THIS BOOK IS NO LONGER THE
PROPERTY OF THE PHILLIPSBURG
FREE PUBLIC LIBRARY

PHILLIPSBURG LIBRARY

6748 9100 041 878 0

D1369977

DATE DUE

6 7 96

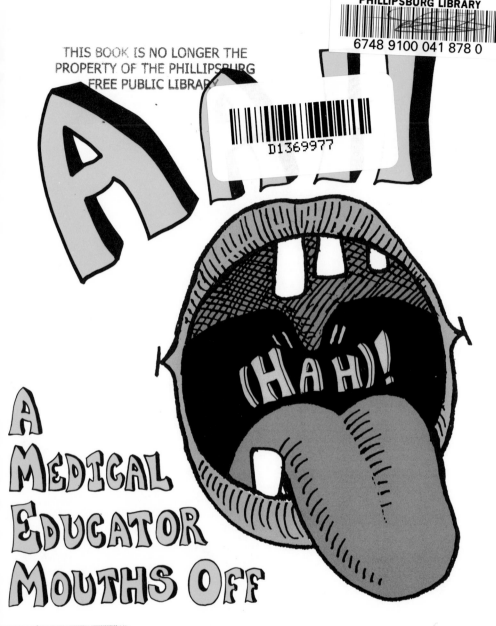

A (HAH)!

A MEDICAL EDUCATOR MOUTHS OFF

Herbert L. Fred, M.D.
Educational Coordinator
HCA Center for Health Excellence
Houston, Texas

ISBN 0-86554-400-X

SAY AAH (HAH)!
Copyright © 1991
Mercer University Press
Macon, Georgia 31207
All rights reserved
Printed in the United States of America

The paper used in this publication meets
the minimum requirements of American National
Standard for Information Sciences—Permanence
of Paper for Printed Library Materials, ANSI Z39.48-1984.

LIBRARY OF CONGRESS CATALOGING-IN-PUBLICATION DATA

Fred, Herbert L.
    Say aah (hah)!: a medical educator mouths off/Herbert L. Fred
    xiv + 156 pp.   15 x 23 cm.   6 x 9″

    Essays previously published in various sources.
    Includes bibliographical references.
    ISBN 0-86554-400-X (alk. paper)
    1. Medicine—Miscellanea. I. Title.
    [DNLM: 1. Medicine—collected works. 2. Medicine—hu-
mor. WZ 7 F852s]
R708.F84   1991
610—dc20
DNLM/DLC   91-27294
for Library of Congress   CIP

CONTENTS

DEDICATION

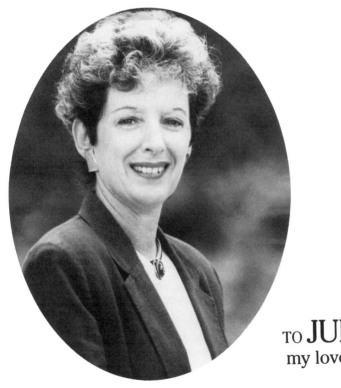

TO JUDY
my lover *(& my wife)*

PHILLIPSBURG LIBRARY
PHILLIPSBURG, N. J.

FOREWORD

We readers last saw Dr. Fred jogging out of his previous book.* That photograph of his run on the Great Wall of China captured something essential: therein we glimpsed a determined man going his way alone, minus any supporting cast. This was a man in touch with his own inner resources, stimulated by the possibilities of the world around him. Taking brief respites in Pithdom to produce these new pearls, Dr. Fred remains a man on the move, dashing out of this book, too.

Having worked with this man for three years, and listening to his voice on the phone nearly every day, I know one thing with eerie certainty: he is the Andy Rooney of the medical world—a Texas straight shooter with emphatic tendencies who keeps the strictest count of the milestones and millstones that give medicine its majesty and muddle. And with a twinkle in his eye, a twinge in his gut, and ten minutes before his next meeting, he can recount most of them to you—entertainingly, eloquently, and with *emphasis.* Luckily for us non-physicians, Dr. Fred's writings also make forays beyond medical issues.

Elephant Medicine—and More: Musings of a Medical Educator (Macon: Mercer University Press, 1988).

As the body jogs, the mind streaks. That has been my experience with Dr. Fred. Whenever he asks, "Can I run such-and-such past you?" I never know whether to expect a blurred form on my doorstep or a FAX in my mail stack. For all the times he has left me standing still, this is one time I got in the race ahead of him—the foreword to his preface. While I gloat, readers should sample this latest Fredian caseload. The essays are pandemically thoughtful and guaranteed to stimulate mental appetites of all kinds (possibly creating a new race of Herb-ivores).

Susan M. Carini
Managing Editor
Mercer University Press

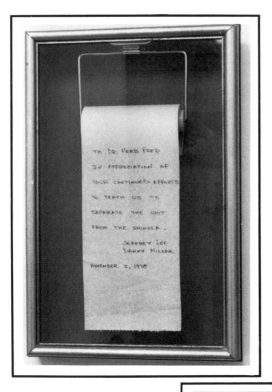

TO DR. HERB FRED
IN APPRECIATION OF
YOUR CONTINUED EFFORTS
TO TEACH US TO
SEPARATE THE SHIT
FROM THE SHINOLA.
JEFFREY LEE
DANNY MILLER
NOVEMBER 2, 1978

THE WHITE HOUSE
WASHINGTON

October 4, 1988

Dear Dr. Fred:

Nancy and I are delighted to join with all those
gathered to congratulate you on your retirement as
Director of Medical Education at St. Joseph Hospital
after 27 years in that field.

Yours has been a career marked by outstanding
dedication and achievement, earning the respect and
admiration of your friends and colleagues alike. We
are happy to share in this special time in your life
and to send our best wishes for good fortune and
happiness in the years ahead.

Again, congratulations on this memorable occasion.

Sincerely,

Ronald Reagan

Dr. Herbert L. Fred
Director of Medical Education
St. Joseph Hospital
Houston, Texas

PREFACE

Of the various diplomas, certificates, awards, and mementos that I proudly display in my office, two are my favorites. One is a personal letter from President Ronald Reagan, commending my dedication to and achievements in the field of medical education. The other is a roll of toilet paper. On the toilet paper is a handwritten note from two medical students: "To Dr. Herb Fred, in appreciation of your continued efforts to teach us to separate the shit from the shinola. —Jeffrey Lee and Danny Miller, November 2, 1978"

Few would question why I treasure my commendation from the president of the United States. But why do I relish that roll of toilet paper? Because it is different, very different, from conventional ways of showing appreciation. More important, it reflects to a tee my philosophy—think for yourself, organize your thoughts carefully, then convey them clearly, succinctly, emphatically, and with honesty. When we do that, we do more than separate shit from shinola. We become leaders, not followers; and we rise above the norm of mediocrity.

That philosophy underpins this book. The essays assembled here offer something "only" for doctors, for mentors, for runners—in fact, for everybody. And in case you're wondering about the title, wonder no longer. "Say aah" is a trademark of my profession; "hah" suggests surprise or joy; and "aha" denotes revelation, surprise, or triumph. So read these essays and say "aah," "hah," or "aha."

H.L.F.

ACKNOWLEDGMENTS

I am indebted to Pat Robie, Rose Marie Morgan, and Dr. Ken Sack for their invaluable critiques of these essays; to Lenore Polk for her typing, proofreading, and general savvy; and to Adie Marks for his wizardly cartoons on the cover and throughout the text.

Special thanks are due Margaret Jordan Brown, Mercer University Press's incomparable book designer. If she could design the human body as proficiently as she designs books, doctors would go out of business.

And speaking of M.D.s, I owe much to Susan Carini, Mercer's peerless and fearless Manuscript Doctor. She always knew when to cut, how to sew, and what to prescribe.

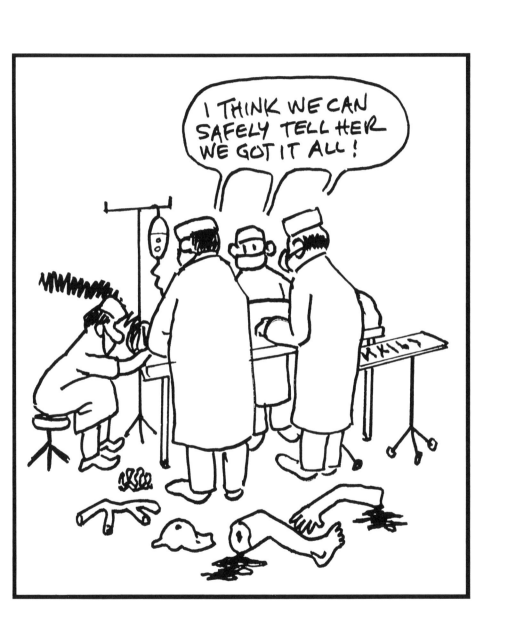

FOR DOCTORS ONLY

There's an awful lot of sin in medicine.

H.L.F.

—in "Medicine or Medisin?"

By moving from the bedside to the laboratory, we are becoming proficient in ordering tests, but deficient in taking a pertinent medical history and doing a good physical examination. As a clinician and as a patient, I find that trade-off uneven and unfortunate.

H.L.F.

—in "The CPC: Historical Considerations, Benefits, and Drawbacks"

MEDICINE OR MEDISIN?*

Medicine. We study it, practice it, prescribe it, buy it, and take it—yet we take its meaning for granted. According to *Webster's,* medicine can be (1) a substance or preparation used in treating disease or (2) the science and art of preventing, alleviating, or curing disease. Sandwiched between these definitions, however, is the one that fits our profession best: something that affects well-being. For no matter how we practice medicine, we affect the well-being of our patients.

In medicine today, quite a few "somethings" affect well-being. Nobody disputes that recent technologic advances have enhanced the potential for good patient care. But these same advances have triggered a spate of indiscriminate, exorbitantly expensive testing and treatment. They have also spawned unrealistic expectations in patients, their families, and even some physicians. Add to all of this the myriad constraints imposed by insurance companies, the incessant pressures created by federally mandated regulations, the glut of "for-profit-not-for-patient" hospital administrators, the lawsuits lurking around every corner, the fraud and deceit in the halls of science, the gobs of paperwork—you get the picture. There's an awful lot of sin in medicine.

*Reprinted by permission from the *Southern Medical Journal* 1990; 83:269.

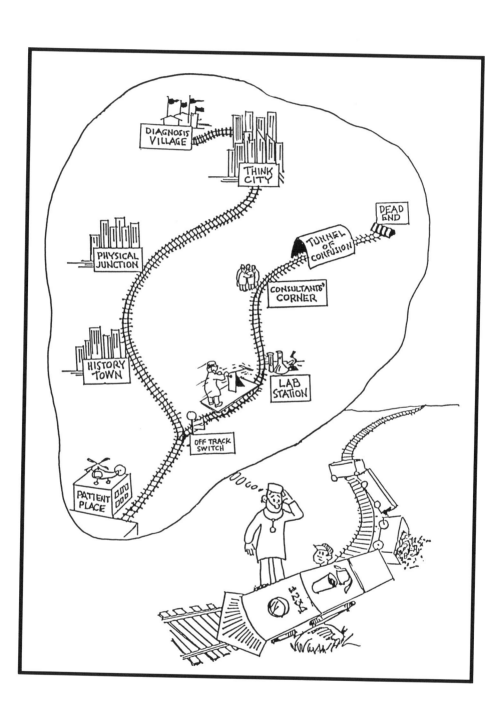

DIAGNOSTIC DERAILMENT*

When you're up to your ears in trouble, try using the part that isn't submerged.

—Quoted by McKenzie[1]

When a person gets sick, a journey begins. Ordinarily, the journey is not solitary: family members and friends join in along the way. And if the sickness persists, a physician usually comes on board. But even in the hands of the most competent physician, the trip to the wellness station may have many detours.

Doctors and trains have several things in common. Both serve the public, both have tight schedules, both run for hours without stopping, and both frequently arrive late. Most important, both may get derailed—one mechanically, the other diagnostically—particularly when they go too fast or fail to heed warning signals.

*Reprinted by permission from the *Southern Medical Journal* 1989; 82:1333.

Similarities between doctors and trains end once derailment occurs. Cognizant or not of derailment, doctors keep right on going, but trains are immediately immobilized, sometimes permanently. Furthermore, doctors can get back on track by their own mental efforts.

What causes diagnostic derailment? Though many articles address this topic, none provides information as insightful and practical as the study Gruver and Freis reported in 1957.[2] In light of the way we practice medicine these days, their findings are even more applicable now. They emphasized that correctable diagnostic errors result not so much from lack of medical knowledge as from deficiencies of medical judgment, alertness, and thoroughness. The deficiencies included failure to (1) obtain an adequate medical history; (2) order routine screening tests, such as blood count, urinalysis, and roentgenogram of the chest; (3) account for symptoms, signs, or laboratory data that do not fit the clinical impression; (4) carry out indicated studies beyond those done initially; (5) recognize new illnesses developing on top of previously established chronic diseases (the prejudiced viewpoint); (6) realize that x-ray examination may not disclose pathologic changes (false-negative results); and (7) review periodically the accumulated data and repeat the physical examination when the illness is prolonged. To this checklist, I would add two other failures—failure to remember that tests and procedures can give false-*positive* results, and failure to appreciate that consultants can be wrong.

During thirty-five years as a full-time medical educator, I have "engineered" my share of diagnostic derailments and have witnessed many others. In every case, the fault has been the same—too much *doing* and not enough *thinking*. Now, when diagnostic derailment seems imminent or, in fact, has already occurred, I return to the previously mentioned checklist. I also ask myself: Could the patient's problem be purely or primarily emotional? Am I dealing with factitious disease? Is the illness one that medical science has not yet specifically identified (e.g., AIDS ten years ago)?

Whether it be health care or rail travel, a smooth journey is never guaranteed. A doctor's diagnostic "switches" can be as prone to failure as switches on a railroad. But derailed trains can't think themselves back on track. Derailed doctors can.

REFERENCES

[1]McKenzie EC (Ed.). *14,000 Quips & Quotes.* New York, Greenwich House, 1984, p. 514.

[2]Gruver RH, Freis ED. A study of diagnostic errors. *Ann Intern Med* 47:108–20, 1957.

SOLICITED EDITORIALS: CREDENCE BY FIAT*

Always believe the expert.
—Virgil
Aeneid, xi, 19 B.C.

Let every eye negotiate for itself and trust no agent.
—Shakespeare
Much Ado about Nothing,
2.1.184

"This study adds nothing to available information."
That statement (or variants thereof) turns up repeatedly in peer reviews of articles submitted to the medical journal I edit. It even appears at times in the medical literature as part of solicited editorials commenting on someone else's work. This type of statement frustrates and irritates me because it is wrong, literally. A study always adds *something* to available

*Reprinted by permission from the *Southern Medical Journal* 1990; 83:734.

information. What the critics presumably mean—but don't say—is that the study adds nothing *worthwhile* to availableinformation. And these same critics often make matters worse by not explaining their reasoning and not recommending ways to correct the alleged deficiencies.

Solicited editorials that critique a particular study have much in common with conventional peer reviews. The two differ primarily in that one is published and the other remains confidential. While the confidential review involves just the critic, the editor, and the author, the published editorial can influence how widely the study gets read and how it is interpreted.

When a solicited editorial zeroes in on another article, it should bring into perspective and expand the substance of that article. Readers deserve no less. An expert's balanced discussion of the issues can be especially instructive if it addresses the appropriateness of the study, the methods used, and the validity, implications, and utility of the results. Yet all too frequently the expert merely rehashes material presented in the study, touches on several tangential topics, and seizes the opportunity to advertise his own contributions to the field.

Granted, a solicited editorial is only an opinion. But it is also a voice of authority, thus creating the potential for credence by fiat—"It must be true because an expert said it." So, the more decisive the opinion, the more circumspect the expert ought to be and the more scrutiny the solicited editorial ought to receive—before and after publication.

DIZZY MEDICAL WRITING: REPORT ON RECENT RELAPSES*

When Dizzy Dean finished his pitching career, he became a popular baseball announcer. The language he used during those broadcasts is now legendary. In remembrance of Old Diz, we created the Dizzy Awards—awards for bewildering, unintentionally comical, or just plain terrible medical writing.[1] The winning excerpts came from prominent medical journals. Soon after we presented the awards, we uncovered many more candidates, making additional awards necessary.[2] The competition was so stiff that ties occurred in some categories.

In our third presentation,[3] we concluded that the memory of Old Diz would be around for a long, long time and that dizzy medical writing would be, too. To support those conclusions, we present the newest honorees.

The Switch Hitter Award

"The cardiac ambulance had been asked to attend him as he had become unconscious in his front garden."
—What did the ambulance say when asked?

The Placed on the Disabled List Award (a tie)

"... optic perineuritis was probably the cause of optic disk

*Reprinted by permission from the *Southern Medical Journal* 1989; 82:897–99.

Patricia Robie is coauthor of this article.—ED.

edema observed in the patients described by Wu and associates and Reik and associates who had normal cerebrospinal fluid pressure and meningitis."

—We hope the doctors recovered from their meningitis.

and

"Early relapse results in presentation to neurologists or paediatricians with epilepsy."

—Would an internist with epilepsy do?

The Cases at the Bat Award

"Only 13 cases have been reported to date in the literature, of which four were pregnant."

—Nine months from now, there should be at least four more cases to report.

The Bad Bounce Award

"The indolent course of this patient's disease may be attributed to the slow invasion of the thyroid by a contiguous tuberculous lymph node."

—Since when can lymph nodes invade thyroids?

The Removed from the Lineup Award (a tie)

"The aim of this study was primarily to determine the importance of death from undiagnosed peptic ulcer complications. . . ."

—Death is generally *very* important, whatever the cause.

and

". . . the patient is potentially resectable."

—Ah, cut it out.

The Who's on First, What's on Second Award

"Though the findings refer to male homosexuals in Stockholm, they are probably also valid for people infected by other routes."

—Is Route 66 infectious?

The Batted Out of Order Award

"The test was regarded as positive when any of the three solutions exactly reproduced the globus symptoms of which they complained."
—Our solutions never complain.

The Out in Left Field Award

"The role of confusion is left to be explained. It explains the relationship between surgical acceptance and the determinants of surgical failure or success."
—We feel *right* in telling you that our confusion is still *left*.

The Caught Napping Award (a tie)

"The TSH response of the 150 patients who underwent TRH stimulation studies also were classified. . . ."
—Were it?

and

"Signs of massive left-sided pleural effusion with contralateral mediastinal shift was also present."
—Was they?

The Wrong Ballpark Award (a tie)

"Observations of muscle enlargement after partial nerve lesions have most commonly been described in the sciatic nerve."
—Next time, try describing them in a medical journal.

and

"Recurrent episodes of *Yersinia* bacteremia have been described in several patients. . . ."
—A few have also been described in the medical literature.

The Questionable Call Award

"Hours after admission, the referring hospital called to report. . . ."

—After we admit a referring hospital, we don't allow it to talk on the phone.

The Three Runs, No Hits, One Error Award

"In three published patients, the fistula originated from the oesophagus. . . ."
—The last patient we published was mashed by the printing press.

The Postponed Because of Wet Grounds Award

"If the diagnosis cannot be made with the above studies and the patient has an active urinary sediment, percutaneous renal biopsy should be considered."
—What if the urinary sediment is sedentary?

The Make-Up Game Award (a tie)

". . . hepatic fibrosis was already present, leading us to consider the possible potentialization of the toxic effect of vitamin A by other unknown factors. . . ."
—The potentiality of finding "potentialization" in the dictionary is not even potentially potent.

and

". . . conditions associated with enterococcal bacteremia in 75 evaluatable patients."
—We have run out of patience trying to evaluate "evaluatable" patients.

The Caught Out of Position Award

"He also had Roth spots, hepatomegaly, and a right middle lobe infiltrate on chest radiography."
—If our chest films covered that much territory, we could throw away our ophthalmoscopes.

The Scouting Report Award (a tie)

". . . cardiac emboli are either extremely rare or have been greatly under-recognized in the HbSS literature."
—We were looking for cardiac emboli in the arteries, not the literature.

and

"Nonetheless, it is interesting that of the four patients who embolized, three did so. . . ."
—Where did the patients embolize to?

The Out at Home Award

"On admission, we were impressed by the widely fluctuating neurologic reactions and progressive hyperthermia."
—To which hospital were you admitted?

The Wrong Pitch Award

". . . the patient was tested for antibodies to the human immunodeficiency virus, but he was negative."
—Since when do tests have gender?

The Time Called Award (a tie)

"Postmortem studies . . . have shown that after sudden death, congestive heart failure is the most frequent mode of death in adults with cardiac sarcoidosis."
—Strange, but we've never seen a case of congestive heart failure that developed *after* death.

and

"A 56-year-old white man was admitted . . . for episodes of syncope and sudden death."
—Exactly how many times did he die?

The Screwball Award

"Rhinoliths are not common but like other rare conditions have an attraction and therefore will be familiar."
—Who nose what that means?

The Balk Award

"Experimental evidence, based on results of radiography and subsequent sagittal sectioning of a frozen, unembalmed human thorax, corroborated the authors' hypothesis that this finding is related to loss of tangential imaging of the apex of the hemidiaphragm due to cephalic angulation of the central beam accompanied by projection of extra-pleural fat onto the base of the left lung."
—Could you expand on that, please?

The Arguing with the Umpire Award

"In contrast to the opinions of some who feel that the glucagon test is outmoded, this patient. . . ."
—Patients always contrast with opinions.

The Debris on the Playing Field Award

"Despite experimental evidence [th]at colchicine, like vincristine, binds to tubulin, the subunit protein of microtubules, with impairment of rapid axoplasmic transport in peripheral nerves and damage to lysosomes and myofilaments in skeletal muscle, reports of colchicine neuropathy and myopathy in man have been limited to a few examples of excessive colchicine self-medication."
—You've gout to be kidding.

The Flagpole Award

". . . liposuction is not indicated for everyone under all circumstances."
—You'll get no argument from us.

The Bag of Soda Pop and Cup of Popcorn Award

"The six patients were not evaluated for tuberculosis until radiology of pulmonary consultations were obtained."
—????

The No Hitter Award

"Besides causing lung damage, our data suggest that. . . ."
—We hope your data carry good malpractice insurance.

The Out of the Ballpark Award

"Two months ago a 3 cm hard mobile parotid tumour disappeared between the ward and theatre."
—Did you look for it behind the door?

The Batty Title Award (four-way tie)

"The Ectopic Kidney in the Emergency Department"
—Unless accompanied by their owners, kidneys should never enter the Emergency Department.

and

"*Mycobacterium chelonae* Causing Otitis Media in an Ear-Nose-and-Throat Practice"
—Did the practice get well or go deaf?

and

"Simple Treatment for Chronic Female Infections"
—If a female infection interacts with a male infection, will a baby infection develop?

and

"Long-Segment Coronary Ulcerations in Survivors of Sudden Cardiac Death"
—Where can we sign up to survive death?

The Hall of Shame Award (a tie)

"Two cases of pulmonary embolism from superior vena caval thrombosis due to a Hickman catheter seen by the authors during a recent two-month period emphasize that this complication is not rare."

—The not-rare complication seen by us in that sentence is the difficulty seeing what was seen by the authors.

and

"During induction, difficulty was encountered in drawing blood from the catheter, which responded on several occasions to urokinase instillation (5,000 U in 2 ml saline)."

—Difficulty was also encountered by us in drawing conclusions from that sentence, which didn't respond on several occasions to re-reading.

REFERENCES

[1]Fred HL, Robie P. Dizzy medical writing. *South Med J* 1983; 76:1165–66.

[2]Fred HL, Robie P. Dizzy medical writing: Part II. *South Med J* 1984; 77:755–56.

[3]Fred HL, Robie P. Dizzy medical writing: Concluded. *South Med J* 1985; 78:1498-1501.

DIZZY MEDICAL WRITING:
WILL IT NEVER END?*

Eight years ago we published the first in a series of articles on dizzy medical writing.[1-4] We had hoped that by drawing attention to such lexical litter we might somehow reduce its frequency and extent. So far, we've failed, but we haven't given up the cause.

Presented here are the most recent winners of the Dizzy Awards. These awards honor the late, great Dizzy Dean and are given for excellence in bewildering, unintentionally comical, or downright terrible medical writing.

The Extra Innings Award (a tie)

"The epicardium, cardiac valves, and endocardium appeared normal. The epicardium, cardiac valves, and endocardium appeared normal."

—But what about the epicardium, cardiac valves, and endocardium?

and

". . . and iodide-induced thyrotoxicosis has been recognized since 1820 by the French physician Coindet."

—Amazing! After 171 years he can still see!

*Reprinted by permission from the *Southern Medical Journal* 1991; 84:755–59.

Patricia Robie is coauthor of this article.—ED.

The Placed on the Disabled List Award

"A 79-year-old non-insulin-dependent diabetic woman presented with severe pain in the rectum and urgency."
—How does pain in the urgency present?

The Caught Out of Position Award (a tie)

"The next study was performed by our group at the University of Southern California, which was published in 1977."
—How do you publish a university?
                              and
"Livido is a term first used to describe a violet discoloration of the skin due to a local circulatory disturbance in the 1860s."
—There's also a disturbance in the syntax of that sentence in the 1990s.

The Screwball Award

"This case points out the continued importance of performing and culturing unusual skin lesions in patients with AIDS."
—How does one perform a skin lesion?

The Touch Every Base Award

"The proposal that cobalt-induced lung disease might thus at least partly result from 'transitional metal overload' leading to oxygen free radical tissue injury, does not appear to have been hitherto envisaged, and such a mechanism is admittedly still speculative, but this hypothesis merits further experimental investigation."
—Perhaps you'd like to qualify that statement?

The Wrong Pitch Award

"A promising prophylaxis for general surgery, although not

yet confirmed, is very low-dose warfarin at 1 mg daily started
3 weeks before elective surgery."
—Good health would work better.

The Scorecard Award

"There were also significant differences between the
average extension of the pleural lesions in the following
groups: cases with glucose lower/higher than 60 mg/dl
(p ⟨ 0.01); pH lower/higher than 7.30 (p ⟨ 0.0003); pH lower/
higher than 7.35 (p ⟨ 0.0002); glucose ⟨ 60 mg/dl plus
pH ⟨ 7.30/glucose ⟩ 60 mg/dl plus pH ⟩ 7.30 (p ⟨ 0.002); and
glucose ⟨ 60 mg/dl plus pH ⟨ 7.35/glucose ⟩ 60 mg/dl plus
pH ⟩ 7.35 (p ⟨ 0.002)."
—That figures, more or less.

The Bag of Soda Pop and Cup of Popcorn Award (a tie)

"In contrast to the Framingham study data, we detected no
clustering of thromboembolic complications."
—"We" and "data" always contrast with one another.
                              and
"There were notable deviations in performance and
interpretation between the nephrologists and the standard
urinalysis."
—Obviously. Urinalyses, standard or otherwise, can't
perform or interpret.

The New Pitch Award

"The level of suspicion for the involvement of *B. fragilis* in
septic arthritis ordinarily is quite low, yet it accounted for 26
(8.6%) of 302 cases of anaerobic joint infection reported in the
literature."
—Is level-of-suspicion-induced arthritis a newly
recognized entity?

The Switch Hitter Award (a tie)

"At referral, ENT examination revealed marked

nasopharyngeal and posterior oropharyngeal lymphoid hypertrophy causing complete post-nasal obstruction was observed."

—We refer patients, not ENT examinations.

and

". . . the pulmonary function studies of our patients revealed a restrictive pattern, and they had only a few complaints despite widespread radiographic changes."

—Our pulmonary function studies never complain.

The Balk Award

"A literature review by Arenberg and McCreary (1971), produced 11 reported cases to which he added three new ones."

—Which he is they?

The No Hits, No Runs, One Error Award (a three-way tie)

"Although they have been well described, the contribution of occupational factors is often overlooked. . . ."

—They is?

and

"The prevalence of these signs are sufficiently low. . . ."

—It are?

and

"Keeping facilities, clothing, and equipment clean are important. . . ."

—Is you certain?

The Caught Napping Award (a three-way tie)

"Human cysticercosis is almost caused by Cysticercus cellulosae."

—What else almost causes it?

and

"Patients who continued to have positive blood culture results while receiving appropriate antibiotic therapy had a poor diagnosis."

—The best therapy for a poor diagnosis is appropriate editing.

and

"The conclusions reached probably depend in part on criteria chose for defining a positive result."
—You chose chose instead of choosing chosen?

The Wild Pitch Award

"The etiology of idiopathic hoarseness is multifactorial. . . ."
—You must know something we don't know.

The Make-Up Game Award (a three-way tie)

"The benefits of pancreatic resection and necrosectomy still require full evaluation."
—Necrosectomy?

and

"In this patient, coronary angiography revealed a large, central cavern fistulating into the left atrium. . . ."
—"Fistulating" isn't in our dictionary.

and

"A 62-year-old man developed a fistula between the right ventricle and the stomach after Thal fundic patching of an emetogenic rupture of the esophagus."
—That emetogenic rupture of our language needs patching, too.

The Pop-Up Award

"The patient reported feeling a 'pop' in his right face while he was eating."
—Well, it's better to have a right face than a wrong face, a left face, or an about-face.

The Collision at Home Plate Award

"Urinalysis was grossly bloody with erythrocytes too numerous to count."
—What caused the urinalysis to bleed?

The Wrong Ball Park Award (a four-way tie)

"In the latter article, the lesions initially appeared as erythematous papulopustules similar to 'swimming pool folliculitis,' but then became bullous and necrotic."
—It's enough for articles to have bad grammar, much less erythematous papulopustules.

and

"A case of neurofibromatosis is reported in a patient. . . ."
—We report our cases in medical journals, never in patients.

and

"Systemic mycotic aneurysms and rare pulmonary mycotic aneurysms in intravenous drug abusers have been reported in intravenous drug abusers.
—Sam, have you read today's *Intravenous Drug Abuser?*

and

"The highest incidence of remote neuromuscular disorders in cancer has previously been reported in lung carcinoma."
—Reports in lung carcinoma are harder to read than are those in medical journals.

The Broken Bat Award

"Although the patient's initial presentation is consistent with psoas abscess, *Streptococcus pneumoniae* is rarely described as a pathogen."
—Please check the line, operator. We have a bad connection.

The Cases at the Bat Award (a tie)

". . . only three of nine cases were sufficiently ill to miss work, none were hospitalized, and two untreated case-patients were asymptomatic."
—When our "cases" are too ill to work, our patients work for them.

and

"Although more case-patients than noncase patients reported a rural residence and out door activities. . . ."

—Casing patients is risky.

The Bad Bounce Award

"Only three cases of CMV pneumonitis presenting with the clinical syndrome of hypoxemia and infiltrates on x-ray film with lung biopsy or autopsy confirmation of CMV cytopathic effect in the absence of other pathogens have been reported, to our knowledge."

—Boy, that road was bumpy!

The Batted Out of Order Award (a tie)

"There is ample evidence that bacteraemia occurs after certain forms of dental treatment, defined as extraction, scaling, and surgery including the gingival tissue by the working party of the British Society for Antimicrobial Chemotherapy."

—One more time, please.

and

"A patient with the acquired immunodeficiency syndrome (AIDS) developed severe cyanosis after bronchoscopy (oxygen saturation 34%) from methaemoglobinaemia."

—Bronchoscopy from methaemoglobinaemia is a serious problem.

The Flag Pole Award (a tie)

"Only surgery offers a reasonable chance of cure for most diseases."

—Ah, cut it out.

and

"Cryptococcosis is unique among opportunistic fungal infections because it is the only disease that can occur in normal individuals."

—Balderdash!

The Hall of Shame Award

"As an outpatient 1 month later the blood pressure was 170/100 mm Hg. . . ."
—Was the blood pressure male or female?

The Word Series Award (a tie)

"Because pleural effusions of unknown origin are frequently caused by malignant tumor, especially bronchogenic carcinoma, fiberoptic bronchoscopy is of value in the diagnostic work-up of a pleural effusion of unknown origin and should be performed early to make a diagnosis of malignancy or other entities, particularly in those patients who have hemoptysis or concurrent pulmonary lesions, such as pulmonary collapse, mass, and consolidation, on their chest x-ray films."
—I think we're lost.

and

"As measurements of coronary reserve after pharmacologic stimulation are impractical for most catheterization laboratories, I believe it is reasonable to conclude that patients with an ischemic electrocardiographic response to exercise, coupled with a limited (less than 5% increase) left ventricular ejection fraction response to exercise, or fall in ejection fraction (to exclude the 'false-positive' electrocardiographic responses to stress), should be suspected of having a cardiac basis for their chest pain syndrome."
—Is that all you've got to say?

The Blooper Award

"This report is comprised of three unusual patients."
—And that sentence is composed of one misuse of "comprise."

The Called on Account of Darkness Award

"We believe, however, that this approach to examining data on high cholesterol concentrations may be of value in highlighting not only points of qualitative uncertainty, such as local prevalences of high cholesterol concentrations and the mortality associated with a given concentration but also, more importantly, points of qualitative uncertainty, such as the long term benefits and risks of treatment that lowers cholesterol concentration and what these are in groups not studied in trials—that is, women and certain age and ethnic groups."
—It's been a long day.

The Out in Left Field Award

"The clinical and pathological findings of five adult cases of idiopathic nonsyndromatic paucity of interlobular bile ducts are reported."
—You said a mouthful, doc.

The Questionable Call Award

"In view of the danger of heparin-induced cardiac tamponade, hemodialysis should not be performed with caution in patients with SLE who have severe, active systemic vasculitis and pericarditis."
—Why not?

The Who's on First, What's on Second Award

"On admission, we were unable to obtain either pulse or blood pressure."
—What hospital were you admitted to?

The Full Count Award

"It is likely that this reflected the close correlational

relationships between clinical and biopsy variables, the strong clinical models generated, and the inclusion in the clinical models of the previously neglected clinical variables, duration of renal disease before biopsy and the presence of vasculitis or comorbid disease."
—Are you sure?

The Peanuts and Cracker Jack Award

"It is possible that the observation of enhanced gastric emptying rates for meals with exercise has clinical application."
—Is the same true for meals with the King of Siam?

The Inserted into the Lineup Award

"The pathologic process of sacroiliac joint inflammation is poorly understood due to the limited number of direct of studies of this joint."
—That sentence is also poorly understood.

The Mix-Up in the Outfield Award

"It appears at present that pathologic changes of sacroiliitis cannot be reorganized at an earlier stage with the use of MRI than with conventional radiography or CT.
—Haven't you recognized that your sentence should be reorganized?

The Removed from the Lineup Award

"Catheter function was preserved in all patients who were completely lysed."
—Isn't it against the law to lyse patients?

The Swing and a Miss Award

"When a woman is diabetic her husband is less likely to

eat the same food as her."
—What does her eat?

The Week Hitter Award

"Cultured material from the previous week revealed coagulase-negative *Staphylococcus aureus....*"
—What part of the week did you culture?

The Batty Title Award (a six-way tie)

"Cerebrospinal Fluid in the Rhinitis Clinic"
—Watch out. The floor is slippery.
and
"Primary and Secondary Hypothyroidism in Nasopharyngeal Carcinoma."
—Did the carcinoma have dry skin, fatigue, and puffy face?
and
"Thyroid Deficiency in the Framingham Study"
—We are skeptical of any study done by cretins.
and
"Motor Vehicle Driving among Diabetics Taking Insulin and Non-diabetics."
—Careful, that's a car full.
and
"Predictive Factors for Bactibilia in Acute Cholecystitis."
—We predict there's no such thing as bactibilia.
and
"Idiopathic Biliary Ductopenia in Adults: A Report of Five Cases."
—Is that the opposite of idiopathic biliary ductocytosis?

REFERENCES

[1]Fred HL, Robie P. Dizzy medical writing. *South Med J* 1983; 76:1165–66.

[2]Fred HL, Robie P. Dizzy medical writing: Part II. *South Med J* 1984; 77:755–56.

[3]Fred HL, Robie P. Dizzy medical writing: Concluded. *South Med J* 1985; 78:1498–1501.

[4]Fred HL, Robie P. Dizzy medical writing: Report on recent relapses. *South Med J* 1989; 82:897–99.

TIA IS A TIA*

What would your diagnosis be if a patient had a focal sensory or motor impairment that came on abruptly, disappeared within twenty-four hours, and left no residua? If your answer is "TIA"—transient ischemic attack—you could be wrong in up to 30% of such cases.[1] And if your diagnosis is wrong, your treatment could be dangerous, and the outcome could be tragic.

Some experts say that tests to confirm TIA do not exist.[1] The reason is obvious. These episodes are so brief and unpredictable that demonstrating focal cerebral hypoperfusion during an actual attack is virtually impossible.[2] Clearly, then, the diagnosis is always *presumptive.* Failure to appreciate this fact stifles consideration of mechanisms other than ischemia and probably explains why articles on this syndrome typically deal with prognosis and pay little or no attention to differential diagnosis.

Over the years I have learned that numerous disorders can mimic TIAs. The more I search for them—at the bedside and in the medical literature—the more of them I find (see Table). And the more of them I find, the more misleading "TIA" becomes.

A few physicians recognize the hazards of the term "TIA" and recommend "TND"—transient neurologic deficit.[12, 16] Yet "deficit" indicates too little of something (such as hypoglycemia), which might discourage one from considering too much of something (such as cocaine). Substituting

*Reprinted by permission from *Houston Medicine* 1989; 5:76–79.

"disturbance" for "deficit" would be an improvement, but if we're set on acronyms, why not use "TNA"—transient neurologic abnormality? Compared with TIA and TND, TNA defines the problem accurately, carries no misguiding implications, thwarts premature and presumptive conclusions, and assures a more thoughtful diagnostic approach.

   TIA is a TIA—Treacherously Inadequate Acronym.

TABLE
DISORDERS WITH MANIFESTATIONS SUGGESTING TRANSIENT ISCHEMIC ATTACKS*

Metabolic
Hypoglycemia[3, 4]
Hypercalcemia[5]
Hypocalcemia[6]
Hyperkalemia[7]
Acute intermittent porphyria[6]

Neoplastic
Hodgkin's disease[8, 9]
Meningioma[10, 11]
Astrocytoma[10, 11]
Glioblastoma[10, 11]
Kaposi's sarcoma[12]
Pheochromocytoma[13]

Infections
Toxoplasmosis[12]
Cryptococcal
   meningoencephalitis[12, 14]
Lyme disease[15]
Tuberculous granulomas of
   the central nervous system[16]

Hematologic
Polycythemia[3, 17]
Extramedullary hematopoiesis[18]

Neuropsychiatric
Hypersensitive carotid sinus
   reflex[19]
Meniere disease[20]
Hysteria[1, 6]
Multiple sclerosis[21-23]
Epilepsy[11]
Hyperventilation[24, 25]
Anxiety[1]

Miscellaneous
Cervical Spondylosis[26]
Migraine[27, 28]
Cerebral amyloidosis[29]
Dural sarcoidosis[30]
Cocaine abuse[31, 32]
Subdural hematoma[10, 33, 34]
Subarachnoid hemorrhage[35]
Volume depletion[1]
Drug reactions[1, 36]

---

*Disorders traditionally linked to TIAs—cardiac dysfunction, embolic disease, and atherosclerosis of the extracranial cerebral vessels—are not included.

REFERENCES

[1]Calanchini PR, Swanson PD, Gotshall RA, et al. Cooperative study of hospital frequency and character of transient ischemic attacks. IV. The reliability of diagnosis. JAMA 1977; 238:2029–33.

[2]Dennis MS, Bamford JM, Sandercock PAG, Warlow CP. Lone bilateral blindness: A transient ischaemic attack. Lancet 1989; 1:185–88.

[3]Millikan CH. The pathogenesis of transient focal cerebral ischemia. Circulation 1965; 32:438–50.

[4]Montgomery BM, Pinner CA. Transient hypoglycemic hemiplegia. Arch Intern Med 1964; 114:680–84.

[5]Longo DL, Witherspoon JM. Focal neurologic symptoms in hypercalcemia. Neurology 1980; 30:200–201.

[6]Fred HL: Unpublished data.

[7]Lee KS, Powell BL, Adams PL. Focal neurologic signs associated with hyperkalemia. South Med J 1984; 77:792–93.

[8]Feldmann E, Posner JB. Episodic neurologic dysfunction in patients with Hodgkin's disease. Arch Neurol 1987; 43:1227–33.

[9]Dulli DA, Levine RL, Chun RW, Dinndorf P. Migrainous neurologic dysfunction in Hodgkin's disease (Letter). Arch Neurol 1987; 44:689.

[10]Ross RT. Transient tumor attacks. Arch Neurol 1983; 40:633–36.

[11]Fisher CM. Transient paralytic attacks of obscure nature: The question of nonconvulsive seizure paralysis. Can J Neurol Sci 1978; 5:267–73.

[12]Engstrom JW, Lowenstein DH, Bredesen DE. Cerebral infarctions and transient neurologic deficits associated with acquired immunodeficiency syndrome. Am J Med 1989; 86:528–32.

[13]Thomas JE, Rooke ED, Kvale WF. The neurologist's experience with pheochromocytoma. A review of 100 cases. JAMA 1966; 197:754–58.

[14]Nowack WJ, Bradsher RW. Cryptococcal meningoencephalitis presenting transient focal cerebral symptoms. South Med J 1989; 82:395–96.

[15]Veenendaal-Hilbers JA, Perquin WVM, Hoogland PH, Doornbos L. Basal meningovasculitis and occlusion of the basilar artery in two cases of Borrelia burgdorferi infection. Neurology 1988; 38:1317–19.

[16]Chari CR, Rao NS. Transient neurologic deficit as a presentation of tuberculosis of the central nervous system. Neurology 1987; 37:1884–85.

[17]Millikan CH, Siekert RG, Whisnant JP. Intermittent carotid and vertebral-basilar insufficiency associated with polycythemia. Neurology 1960; 10:188–96.

[18]Ginsberg AH. Extramedullary hematopoiesis presenting as a transient ischemic attack. Arch Neurol 1985; 42:1020–21.

[19]Uesu CT, Eisenman JI, Stemmer EA. The problem of dizziness and syncope in old age: Transient ischemic attacks versus hypersensitive carotid sinus reflex. J Am Geriatrc Soc 1976; 24:126–35.

[20]Brust JCM. Transient ischemic attacks: Natural history and anticoagulation. *Neurology* 1977; 27:701–707.

[21]Osterman PO, Westerberg C-E. Paroxysmal attacks in multiple sclerosis. *Brain* 1975; 98:189–202.

[22]Twomey JA, Espir MLE. Paroxysmal symptoms as the first manifestations of multiple sclerosis. *J Neurol Neurosurg Psychiatry* 1980; 43:296–304.

[23]Zeldowicz L. Paroxysmal motor episodes as early manifestations of multiple sclerosis. *Can Med Assoc J* 1961; 84:937–41.

[24]Tavel ME. Hyperventilation syndrome with unilateral somatic symptoms. *JAMA* 1964; 187:301–303.

[25]Blau JN, Wiles CM, Solomon FS. Unilateral somatic symptoms due to hyperventilation. *Br Med J* 1983; 286:1108.

[26]Sheehan S. Syndromes of basilar and carotid artery insufficiency: Diagnosis and medical therapy. *South Med J* 1961; 54:465–70.

[27]Levy DE. Transient CNS deficits: A common, benign syndrome in young adults. *Neurology* 1988; 38:831–36.

[28]Fisher CM. Late-life migraine accompaniments as a cause of unexplained transient ischemic attacks. *Can J Neurol Sci* 1980; 7:9–17.

[29]Smith DB, Hitchcock M, Philpott PJ. Cerebral amyloid angiopathy presenting as transient ischemic attacks. *J Neurosurg* 1985; 63:963–64.

[30]Sethi KD, El Gammal T, Patel BR, Swift TR. Dural sarcoidosis presenting with transient neurologic symptoms. *Arch Neurol* 1986; 43:595–97.

[31]Lowenstein DH, Massa SM, Rowbotham MC, *et al.* Acute neurologic and psychiatric complications associated with cocaine abuse. *Am J Med* 1987; 83:841–46.

[32]Mody CK, Miller BL, McIntyre HB, *et al.* Neurologic complications of cocaine abuse. *Neurology* 1988; 38:1189–93.

[33]Herskowitz A, Morrison G. Chronic subdural hematoma with attacks resembling transient ischemia (*Letter*). *Arch Neurol* 1982; 39:740.

[34]Russell NA, Goumnerova L, Atack EA, *et al.* Chronic subdural hematoma mimicking transient ischemic attacks. *J Trauma* 1985; 25:1113–14.

[35]Edwards A, London N, Heagerty AM, *et al.* Aneurysm of anterior communicating artery masquerading as Adams-Stokes disease. *Br Med J* 1984; 289:370–71.

[36]Purvin VA, Dunn DW. Nitrate-induced transient ischemic attacks. *South Med J* 1981; 74:1130–31.

ON NOT KEEPING YOUR MOUTH SHUT*

By examining the tongue of the patient, physicians find out the diseases of the body, and philosophers the diseases of the mind.[1]

We've all heard the saying, "If you want to stay out of trouble, keep your mouth shut." That's good advice for fish and healthy people. But for people who are sick, careful oral examination by an informed physician may be all it takes to establish the diagnosis, even when the patient has no complaints concerning the mouth.

In this report, I draw attention to oral manifestations of *systemic* disease, grouping them according to where they usually appear in the mouth. I make no attempt to include all such lesions or to elaborate on the ones I mention. I do, however, cite appropriate references.

• **LIPS:** Among the telltale markers are telangiectases of Osler-Weber-Rendu disease,[2] brownish-black or blue-gray

*Reprinted by permission from *Houston Medicine* 1990; 6:2–8.

spots of Peutz-Jeghers syndrome,[2, 3] thickened enlargement of acromegaly[4] and hypothyroidism,[5] chancres of syphilis,[6, 7] nodules of metastatic neoplasms,[8] and diffuse, lumpy neuromas associated with pheochromocytoma and medullary carcinoma of the thyroid.[2]

• **TEETH:** Brownish mottling is typical of fluorosis;[9] a red hue is characteristic of erythropoietic porphyria,[10] and a green tint suggests erythroblastosis fetalis.[11] Stunted and peg-shaped upper central incisors (Hutchinson's teeth) and first molars with maldeveloped cusps and a mulberry-like surface (Moon's molars) signal congenital syphilis.[12]

• **GUMS:** Striking hypertrophy with or without friability and easy bleeding may herald scurvy,[13] sarcoidosis,[14] Crohn's disease,[15, 16] amyloidosis,[17] acute leukemia,[18] lymphoma,[19] or Kaposi's sarcoma.[20] Hypertrophy with a strawberry appearance is classic for Wegener's granulomatosis.[21, 22] Progressive brownish-black discoloration may indicate adrenal insufficiency[23, 24] or the melanosis of metastatic melanoma.[25] Dark lines at the gingival margins suggest exposure to heavy metals.[26] The gums can appear lumpy from metastatic neoplasms;[27] be swollen in pemphigus vulgaris;[28] contain fibrous growths in tuberous sclerosis;[2] and show desquamation, ulceration, and extreme redness in mucous membrane pemphigoid.[29] Necrotizing gingivitis progressing rapidly to gangrenous stomatitis is a newly recognized complication of human immunodeficiency virus infection.[30, 31]

• **BUCCAL MUCOSA:** Major findings are the blisters of pemphigus,[32, 33] Koplik spots of measles,[34, 35] angiokeratomata of Fabry's disease,[36, 37] mucous patches of secondary syphilis,[6,7] parchmentlike dryness of Sjögren's syndrome,[38] and the pigmented spots of Peutz-Jeghers syndrome.[3] Unexplained candidiasis (thrush) can be the initial sign of the acquired immunodeficiency syndrome.[39]

• **PALATE:** Located here are the vascularlike, exophytic or flat lesions of Kaposi's sarcoma;[20, 40] other metastatic neoplasms;[41] the cobblestone abnormalities of rhinoscleroma;[42-44] ulcero-nodular changes of leprosy;[6, 45] blue-gray pigmentation of hemochromatosis;[46] and perforations resulting from midline granuloma[47] and syphilitic gumma.[6, 7, 45] Petechiae confined to this part of the mouth, but also evident elsewhere on the body, suggest Korean hemorrhagic fever[48] or parvovirus disease.[49] By contrast, petechiae restricted to the palate alone are a clue to infectious mononucleosis.[50, 51]

• **TONGUE:** Gross enlargement usually means amyloidosis,[52, 53] hypothyroidism,[54, 55] or acromegaly;[4, 55, 56] it occasionally reflects pemphigus[28] or sarcoidosis.[57] Papillary atrophy, with or without pain and redness, suggests vitamin deficiency.[58] Lingual infarction is a feature of temporal arteritis;[59] lumps may be metastatic neoplasm,[60] neuromas,[2] or cysticercosis;[61] and ulcero-nodular changes can signify tuberculosis.[55, 62] Telangiectases of Osler-Weber-Rendu disease commonly involve the anterior part of the tongue,[2] but the hemangiomas of Blue Rubber Bleb Nevus syndrome can affect any part.[63-65] Hairy leukoplakia, a grayish-white corrugated lesion, typically appears on the lateral borders of the tongue as an early sign of infection with the human immunodeficiency virus.[66] Enlarged sublingual salivary glands may denote hypothyroidism.[67]

• **TONSILS:** A yellow-orange or tangerine appearance is pathognomonic of Tangier disease (familial high-density lipoprotein deficiency).[68] Tonsillar masses may be the first sign of sarcoidosis[69] or metastatic neoplasm.[70] Tonsillitis can be the presenting manifestation of typhoid fever,[71] syphilis,[72] leishmaniasis,[73] infectious mononucleosis,[74] and suppurative thrombophlebitis of the internal jugular vein.[75]

• **ORAL ULCERS:** Most oral ulcers are transient, resolve spontaneously, and have no definite connection with systemic disease.[76] When persistent, however, ulcerative lesions in the mouth may be the first or only manifestation of a serious underlying disorder. Such ulcers can arise anywhere in the oral cavity and vary widely in size and shape. They ordinarily represent infection, *e.g.,* histoplasmosis,[77] leishmaniasis,[78, 79] tuberculosis (typical[62] and atypical[80]), cryptococcosis,[81] syphilis,[7] or blastomycosis (South American[82] and North American[83]). Occasionally they represent disseminated neoplasm,[84, 85] Wegener's granulomatosis,[22, 86] Crohn's disease,[87, 88] or scurvy.[89] Recurrent orogenital ulceration suggests Behçet's disease.[90, 91]

Comment

Some of these findings are virtually diagnostic from inspection alone (*e.g.,* telangiectases and tangerine tonsils). Some may require biopsy or culture for precise diagnosis (*e.g.,* hypertrophied gums; ulcers; various lumps and bumps). And some are primarily signals to look for associated clues elsewhere in the body (*e.g.,* possible angiokeratomata should prompt immediate examination of the bathing trunk area, where cutaneous lesions of Fabry's disease are most prominent).

More than an entrance for food and an exit for sound, the mouth can provide quick solutions to sometimes puzzling diagnostic problems. So when you're sick and want to stay out of trouble, don't keep your mouth shut!

REFERENCES

[1]St. Justin (100?–165?), quoted by Strauss MB (Ed). *Familiar Medical Quotations.* Boston, Little, Brown and Company, 1968, pp. 94–95.

[2]Gorlin RJ, Sedano HO. Oral manifestations of systemic genetic disorders (in four parts). *Postgrad Med* 1971; 49: (Jan)144–50, (Feb)159–64, (Mar)155–58, and (Apr)155–60.

[3]Godard JE, Dodds WJ, Phillips JC, Scanlon GT. Peutz-Jeghers syndrome: Clinical and roentgenographic features. *AJR* 1971; 113:316–24.

[4]Roth J, Glick SM, Cuatrecasas P, Hollander CS. Acromegaly and other disorders of growth hormone secretion. Combined clinical staff conference at the National Institutes of Health. *Ann Intern Med* 1967; 66:760–88.

[5]DeGowin EL, DeGowin RL. *Bedside Diagnostic Examination, 2nd Edition.* London, The Macmillan Company, 1969, p. 135.

[6]Shklar G. Oral reflections of infectious diseases (in two parts). *Postgrad Med* 1971; 49:(Jan) 87–92, (Feb) 147–52.

[7]Meyer I, Shklar G. The oral manifestations of acquired syphilis. A study of eighty-one cases. *Oral Surg* 1967; 23:45–57.

[8]Lee BM. Metastasis of colon carcinoma to the lip (*Letter*). *Arch Dermatol* 1972; 105:608.

[9]Singh A, Jolly SS, Bansal BC, Mathur CC. Endemic fluorosis: Epidemiological, clinical and biochemical study of chronic fluorine intoxication in Punjab (India). *Medicine* 1963; 42:229–46.

[10]Wintrobe MM, Lee GR, Boggs DR, *et al. Clinical hematology, 7th Edition.* Philadelphia, Lea & Febiger, 1974, p. 1022.

[11]Witkop CJ Jr, Wolf RO. Hypoplasia and intrinsic staining of enamel following tetracycline therapy. *JAMA* 1963; 185:1008–11.

[12]Harcourt B. Oral disorders associated with ocular disease, II. *Br J Ophthalmol* 1967; 51:284–85.

[13]Chazan JA, Mistilis SP. The pathophysiology of scurvy. A report of seven cases. *Am J Med* 1963; 34:350–58.

[14]Hayter JP, Robertson JM. Sarcoidosis presenting as gingivitis. *Br Med J* 1988; 296:1504.

[15]Bottomley WK, Giorgini GL, Julienne CH. Oral extension of regional enteritis (Crohn's disease). *Oral Surg* 1972; 34:417–20.

[16]Estrin HM, Hughes RW Jr. Oral manifestations in Crohn's disease: Report of a case. *Am J Gastroenterol* 1985; 80:352–54.

[17]Schwartz HC, Olson DJ. Amyloidosis: A rational approach to diagnosis by intraoral biopsy. *Oral Surg* 1975; 39:837–43.

[18]Sinn CM, Dick FW. Monocytic leukemia. *Am J Med* 1956; 20:588–602.

[19]Swanson DL, Kim NK, Theologides A. Burkitt's lymphoma in a 76-year-old woman with diffuse gingival enlargement (*Letter*). *Arch Intern Med* 1978; 138:1581.

[20]Silverman S Jr, Migliorati CA, Lozada-Nur F, *et al.* Oral findings in people with or at high risk for AIDS: A study of 375 homosexual males. *J Am Dent Assoc* 1986; 112:187–92.

[21]Cohen PS, Meltzer JA. Strawberry gums. A sign of Wegener's granulomatosis. *JAMA* 1981; 246:2610–11.

[22]Handlers JP, Waterman J, Abrams AM, Melrose RJ. Oral features of Wegener's granulomatosis. *Arch Otolaryngol* 1985; 111:267–70.

[23]Izzo AJ. Treatment of Addison's disease. *GP* 1955; 12:79–88.

[24]Becker KL, Randall RV. Pigmentation as the presenting feature of Addison's disease: Report of a case. *Metabolism* 1963; 12:1057–62.

[25]Trueblood DV. Malignant melanoma with generalized skin blackening. The white girl who turned black. *Northwest Med* 1947; 46:199–202.

[26]Adour KK. Oral manifestations of systemic disease. *Med Clin North Am* 1966; 50:361–69.

[27]Rentschler RE, Thrasher TV. Gingival and mandibular metastases from rectal adenocarcinoma: Case report and 20 year review of the English literature. *Laryngoscope* 1982; 92:795–98.

[28]Milgraum SS, Kanzler MH, Waldinger TP, Wong RC. Macroglossia. An unusual presentation of pemphigus vulgaris. *Arch Dermatol* 1985; 121:1328–29.

[29]Shklar G, McCarthy PL. Oral lesions of mucous membrane pemphigoid. A study of 85 cases. *Arch Otolaryngol* 1971; 93:354–64.

[30]Editorial: Orofacial manifestations of HIV infection. *Lancet* 1988; 1:976–77.

[31]Winkler JR, Murray PA, Hammerle C. Gangrenous stomatitis in AIDS (*Letter*). *Lancet* 1989; 2:108.

[32]Wood NK, Goaz PW. *Differential Diagnosis of Oral Lesions, 3rd Edition.* St. Louis, The C. V. Mosby Company, 1985, pp. 273–74.

[33]Grattan CEH, Scully C. Oral ulceration: a diagnostic problem. *Br Med J* 1986; 292:1093–94.

[34]Suringa DWR, Bank LJ, Ackerman AB. Role of measles virus in skin lesions and Koplik's spots. *N Engl J Med* 1970; 283:1139–42.

[35]Brem J. Koplik spots for the record. An illustrated historical note. *Clin Pediatr* 1972; 11:161–63.

[36]Fessas P, Wintrobe MM, Cartwright GE. Angiokeratoma corporis diffusum universale (Fabry). First American report of a rare disorder. *Arch Intern Med* 1955; 95:469–81.

[37]Wise D, Wallace HJ, Jellinek EH. Angiokeratoma corporis diffusum. A clinical study of eight affected families. *Q J Med* 1962; 31:177–206.

[38]Cummings NA. Oral manifestations of connective tissue disease. *Postgrad Med* 1971; 49:134–42.

[39]Klein RS, Harris CA, Small CB, *et al.* Oral candidiasis in high-risk patients as the initial manifestation of the acquired immunodeficiency syndrome. *N Engl J Med* 1984; 311:354–58.

[40]Epstein JB, Lozada-Nur F, McLeod WA, Spinelli J. Oral Kaposi's sarcoma in acquired immunodeficiency syndrome: Review of management and report of the efficacy of intralesional vinblastine. *Cancer* 1989; 64:2424–30.

[41]Susan LP, Daughtry JD, Stewart BH, Straffon RA. Palatal metastases in renal cell carcinoma. *Urology* 1979; 13:304–305.

[42]Shum TK, Whitaker CW, Meyer PR. Clinical update on rhinoscleroma. *Laryngoscope* 1982; 92:1149–56.

[43]Lenis A, Ruff T, Diaz JA, Ghandour EG. Rhinoscleroma. *South Med J* 1988; 81:1580–82.

[44]Stiernberg CM, Clark WD, Quinn FB, Bailey BJ. Rhinoscleroma. *Tex Med* 1985; 81:43–46.

[45]Brown RB, Clinton D. Vesicular and ulcerative infections of the mouth and oropharynx. *Postgrad Med* 1980; 67:107–16.

[46]Beitman RG, Frost SS, Roth JLA. Oral manifestations of gastrointestinal disease. *Dig Dis Sci* 1981; 26:741–47.

[47]Fauci AS, Johnson RE, Wolff SM. Radiation therapy of midline granuloma. *Ann Intern Med* 1976; 84:140–47.

[48]International Notes: Korean hemorrhagic fever. *MMWR* 1988; 37:87–96.

[49]Naides SJ, Piette W, Veach LA, Argenyi Z. Human parvovirus B19-induced vesiculopustular skin eruption. *Am J Med* 1988; 84:968–72.

[50]Shiver CB Jr, Frenkel EP. Palatine petechiae, an early sign in infectious mononucleosis. *JAMA* 1956; 161:592–94.

[51]Hoagland RJ. The clinical manifestations of infectious mononucleosis. A report of two hundred cases. *Am J Med Sci* 1960; 240:21–28.

[52]Kyle RA, Bayrd ED. Amyloidosis: Review of 236 cases. *Medicine* 1975; 54:271–99.

[53]Kyle RA, Greipp PR. Amyloidosis (AL). Clinical and laboratory features in 229 cases. *Mayo Clin Proc* 1983; 58:665–83.

[54]Watanakunakorn C, Hodges RE, Evans TC. Myxedema. A study of 400 cases. *Arch Intern Med* 1965; 116:183–90.

[55]Merril A, Kruger GO. An atlas of the tongue. *Am Fam Phys* 1973; 8:158–65.

[56]Dujovny M, Osgood CP, Segal R. Acute acromegalic dyspnea. *Laryngoscope* 1976; 86:1397–1401.

[57]Tillman HH, Taylor RG, Carchidi JE. Sarcoidosis of the tongue. *Oral Surg* 1966; 21:190–95.

[58]Dreizen S. Systemic significance of glossitis. Decoding the tongue's medical messages. *Postgrad Med* 1984; 75:207–15.

[59]Bowdler DA, Knight JR. Lingual claudication and necrosis as a complication of giant cell arteritis. *J Laryngol Otol* 1985; 99:417–20.

[60]Kim RY, Perry SR, Levy DS. Metastatic carcinoma to the tongue. A report of two cases and a review of the literature. *Cancer* 1979; 43:386–89.

[61]Jain RK, Gupta OP, Aryya NC. Cysticercosis of the tongue. *J Laryngol Otol* 1989; 103:1227–28.

[62]Oppenheim H, Livingston CS, Nixon JW, Miller CD. Streptomycin therapy in oral tuberculosis. *Arch Otolaryngol* 1950; 52:910–29.

[63]Baiocco FA, Gamoletti R, Negri A, Rognoni S. Blue rubber bleb nevus syndrome: A case with predominantly ENT localization. *J Laryngol Otol* 1984; 98:317–19.

[64]Jennings M, Ward P, Maddocks JL. Case report: Blue rubber bleb naevus disease: an uncommon cause of gastrointestinal tract bleeding. *Gut* 1988; 29:1408–12.

[65]Hoffman T, Chasko S, Safai B. Association of blue rubber bleb nevus syndrome with chronic lymphocytic leukemia and hypernephroma. *Johns Hopkins Med J* 1978; 142:91–94.

[66]Samaranayake LP, Pindborg JJ. Hairy leucoplakia. Three quarters of patients develop AIDS in two to three years. *Br Med J* 1989; 298:270–71.

[67]Fulop M. Pouting sublinguals: Enlarged salivary glands in myxoedema. *Lancet* 1989; 2:550–51.

[68]Schoenberg BS, Schoenberg DG. Eponym: Tangerine tonsils in Tangier: High-density lipoprotein deficiency. *South Med J* 1978; 71:453–54.

[69]Altug H, Tahsinoglu M, Çelikoğlu S. A case of tonsillar localization of sarcoidosis. *J Laryngol Otol* 1973; 87:417–21.

[70]Monforte R, Ferrer A, Montserrat JM, *et al.* Bronchial adenocarcinoma presenting as a lingual tonsillar metastasis. *Chest* 1987; 92:1122–23.

[71]Johnson PC, Sabbaj J. Typhoid tonsillitis. *JAMA* 1980; 244:362.

[72]Viers Wa. Primary syphilis of the tonsil: Presentation of four cases. *Laryngoscope* 1981; 91:1507–11.

[73]Laudadio P. A case of tonsillar leishmaniasis. *J Laryngol Otol* 1984; 98:213–16.

[74]Aronson MD, Komaroff AL, Pass TM, *et al.* Heterophil antibody in adults with sore throat. Frequency and clinical presentation. *Ann Intern Med* 1982; 96:505–508.

[75]Sinave CP, Hardy GJ, Fardy PW. The Lemierre syndrome: Suppurative thrombophlebitis of the internal jugular vein secondary to oropharyngeal infection. *Medicine* 1989; 68:85–94.

[76]Weingarten NM. Oral ulcers: A diagnostic approach. *Houston Med J* 1986; 2:17–24.

[77]Bennett DE. Histoplasmosis of the oral cavity and larynx. A clinicopathologic study. *Arch Intern Med* 1967; 120:417–27.

[78]Singer C, Armstrong D, Jones TC, Spiro RH. Imported mucocutaneous leishmaniasis in New York City. Report of a patient treated with amphotericin B. *Am J Med* 1975; 59:444–47.

[79]Zinneman HH, Hall WH, Wallace FG. Leishmaniasis of the larynx. Report of a case and its confusion with histoplasmosis. *Am J Med* 1961; 31:654–58.

[80]Volpe F, Schwimmer A, Barr C. Oral manifestation of disseminated *Mycobacterium avium intracellulare* in a patient with AIDS. *Oral Surg* 1985; 60:567–70.

[81]Glick M, Cohen SG, Cheney RT, *et al.* Oral manifestations of disseminated *Cryptococcus neoformans* in a patient with acquired immunodeficiency syndrome. *Oral Surg* 1987; 64:454–59.

[82]Londero AT, Ramos CD. Paracoccidioidomycosis. A clinical and mycologic study of forty-one cases observed in Santa Maria, RS, Brazil. *Am J Med* 1972; 52:771–75.

[83]Bell WA, Gamble J, Garrington GE. North American blastomycosis with oral lesions. *Oral Surg* 1969; 28:914–23.

[84]Wood NK, Goaz PW. *Differential Diagnosis of Oral Lesions, 3rd Edition.* St. Louis, The C. V. Mosby Company, 1985, pp. 133–35.

[85]Voelkerding KV, Sandhaus LM, Kim HC, *et al.* Plasma cell malignancy in the acquired immune deficiency syndrome. Association with Epstein-Barr virus. *Am J Clin Pathol* 1989; 92:222–28.

[86]Fauci AS, Haynes BF, Katz P, Wolff SM. Wegener's granulomatosis: Prospective clinical and therapeutic experience with 85 patients for 21 years. *Ann Intern Med* 1983; 98:76–85.

[87]Varley EWB. Crohn's disease of the mouth. Report of three cases. *Oral Surg* 1972; 33:570–78.

[88]Schiller KFR, Golding P-L, Peebles RA, Whitehead R. Crohn's disease of the mouth and lips. *Gut* 1971; 12:864–65.

[89]Ferguson MM, Dagg JH. Oral ulceration due to ascorbic-acid deficiency (*Letter*). *Lancet* 1974; 1:164.

[90]Chajek T, Fainaru M. Behçet's disease. Report of 41 cases and a review of the literature. *Medicine* 1975; 54:179–96.

[91]James DG. "Silk Route disease" (Behçet's disease). *West J Med* 1988; 148:433–37.

ENIGMATIC ASCITES:
THE FORGOTTEN FOUR*

When ascites is the first, the only, or the predominant sign of fluid retention, the doctor should administer thyroid hormone, strip the pericardium, or open the abdomen!

Absurd as that statement may seem, I devised it as a guide to the four causes of ascites that are curable, but which go *unrecognized* with disconcerting frequency. These "forgotten four" are hypothyroidism; constrictive pericarditis; pancreatitis, usually with pseudocyst formation; and tuberculous peritonitis.

Hypothyroidism: A good physical examination is crucial to the early recognition of myxedema ascites. By the time ascites becomes prominent, better-known and more-frequent signs of hypothyroidism are virtually always present. I have seen nine patients with myxedema ascites, each of whom displayed a

*Reprinted by permission from *Houston Medicine* 1989; 5:2-5.

puffy face; low-pitched voice; slow, slurred speech; dry skin; and, most important, pseudomyotonic deep tendon reflexes. Yet, despite such tell-tale findings, these patients were misdiagnosed, some for years, as having refractory myocardial failure, hepatic cirrhosis, or malignancy.

Failure to recognize hypothyroidism as the cause of ascites can be devastating. Some victims have had a total of 200 paracenteses before the true nature of their illness became evident.[1] Others have undergone one or more exploratory celiotomies.[1,2] One patient had 460 liters of peritoneal fluid removed over a six-year span.[3] And another had six prolonged hospitalizations and extensive investigations for cancer, infection, and liver disease before he died, untreated, from myxedema coma.[4]

Thyroid function studies are indicated, therefore, in every patient with unexplained ascites. As with any test, the results may be at variance with the clinical impression. So the best test is the patient's clinical response to thyroid hormone replacement therapy.

Constrictive pericarditis: This disorder commonly masquerades as hepatic cirrhosis or abdominal carcinomatosis, chiefly because it produces hepatomegaly, various degrees of icterus, and gross ascites with little or no peripheral edema.[5] A careful examination of the neck veins should prevent any diagnostic error. In patients with pericardial constriction, the central venous pressure is elevated and the neck veins typically are distended. By contrast, in patients with hepatic cirrhosis or metastatic malignancy, the central venous pressure is normal and the neck veins are flat.[6] Distinguishing between constrictive pericarditis and restrictive cardiomyopathy can be difficult and occasionally requires exploratory thoracotomy to settle the issue.[7] Regardless, constrictive pericarditis may be cured by stripping the pericardium.[8]

Pancreatitis: Patients with pancreatic ascites characteristically have massive accumulation of free intra-abdominal fluid, often without pain; lose appreciable amounts of weight; and appear chronically ill. Not surprisingly, therefore, the clinical picture mimics that of hepatic cirrhosis, tuberculous peritonitis, or cancer. But in pancreatic ascites, the ascitic fluid amylase content is always markedly elevated, frequently into the thousands.[9] The ascitic fluid protein and serum amylase concentrations are also high in most cases. Occasionally, the fluid is bloody.[10]

In about two-thirds of these patients, the ascites results from a leaking pancreatic pseudocyst; disruption of the pancreatic duct is responsible in the remainder.[11] Though medical management is sometimes effective, most of the patients require surgical intervention to seal the pancreatic leak. Preoperative endoscopic retrograde cholangiopancreatography is valuable in demonstrating the ductal anatomy and site of leakage.[12]

Tuberculous peritonitis: Of the curable types of ascites, this can be the hardest to identify. The two big pitfalls in making the diagnosis are failure to consider the disease and the variable nature of the ascitic fluid. Contrary to popular belief, the fluid may be physically, chemically, microscopically, and bacteriologically normal.[13] Only rarely is it bloody.[13, 14] Stains and cultures often give negative results.[15, 16] Consequently, multiple biopsy specimens of the peritoneum—obtained at laparoscopy[17] or at celiotomy[18]—are often necessary to confirm or exclude tuberculous peritonitis.

These four diseases deserve automatic consideration in every patient with persistent or recurrent ascites, except perhaps in patients with widespread or terminal cancer. This strategy can be particularly rewarding when the patient already has, or is presumed to have, a disease known to cause intractable ascites. I have observed, for example, nine patients with histologically proven hepatic cirrhosis whose long-standing ascites resolved permanently following treatment for coexisting disease—pancreatitis with pseudocyst formation in four, tuberculous peritonitis in two, hypothyroidism in two, and constrictive pericarditis in one.

Tests to determine whether the fluid is a transudate or exudate are neither sensitive nor specific. In fact, hepatic cirrhosis can produce an exudate;[19-22] tuberculous peritonitis often gives a transudate;[13] and hypothyroidism,[1] as well as cancer,[22-24] can generate either a transudate or an exudate.

The results of cytologic studies of ascitic fluid are not always diagnostic and may be misleading. True positives appear in about half of the patients known to have neoplasms.[23, 25] The false positive rate, however, ranges up to 3%.[26] These false positives can occur in patients with hepatic cirrhosis,[25] but they also occur in patients with *curable* causes of ascites such as tuberculosis[27] and pancreatitis.[9]

Percutaneous liver biopsy may preclude further work-up if it discloses cancer or amyloid. But finding cirrhosis or normal tissue will not exclude concomitant pancreatitis, tuberculous peritonitis, hypothyroidism, constrictive pericarditis, or intra- or extrahepatic malignancy.

Finally, this: Routine blood count, urine protein determination, stool guaiac test, serum bilirubin concentration, and plain films of the chest and abdomen can suggest, but never prove, the cause of ascites. Similarly, liver-function tests, gastrointestinal x-ray examination, liver-spleen scan, abdominal ultrasonography, CT scan, and MRI can provide important diagnostic clues, but they never prove the cause of ascites.

In summary: If I have been successful here, my opening statement should no longer seem absurd:

When ascites is the first, the only, or the predominant sign of fluid retention, the doctor should administer thyroid hormone, strip the pericardium, or open the abdomen.

REFERENCES

[1]Dickson J, Natelson EA, Fred HL. Myxedema ascites. *Am Fam Physician* 1970; 1:93.

[2]Baker A, Kaplan M, Wolfe H. Central congestive fibrosis of the liver in myxedema ascites. *Ann Intern Med* 1972; 77:927–29.

[3]Kocen RS, Atkinson M. Ascites in hypothyroidism. *Lancet* 1963; 1:527–30.

[4]Kinney EL. Myxedema ascites. *Am Fam Physician* 1987; 36:134.

[5]Hancock EW. Constrictive pericarditis: Clinical clues to diagnosis. *JAMA* 1975; 232:176–77.

[6]Hirschmann JV. Pericardial constriction. *Am Heart J* 1978; 96:110–22.

[7]Editorial: Restrictive cardiomyopathy or constrictive pericarditis. *Lancet* 1987; 2:372–74.

[8]Kilman JW, Bush CA, Wooley CF, *et al.* The changing spectrum of pericardiectomy for chronic pericarditis: Occult constrictive pericarditis. *J Thorac Cardiovasc Surg* 1977; 74:668–73.

[9]Cameron JL. Chronic pancreatic ascites and pancreatic pleural effusions. *Gastroenterology* 1978; 74:134–40.

[10]Jensen NM, Babior BM. Ascites due to chronic pancreatitis. *JAMA* 1967; 201:228–29.

[11]Sankaran S, Walt AJ. Pancreatic ascites: Recognition and management. *Arch Surg* 1976; 111:430–34.

[12]Davis RE, Graham DY. Pancreatic ascites: The role of endoscopic pancreatography. *Dig Dis* 1975; 20:977–80.

[13]Burack WR, Hollister RM. Tuberculous peritonitis: A study of forty-seven proved cases encountered by a general medical unit in twenty-five years. *Am J Med* 1960; 28:510–23.

[14]Natelson EA, Allen TW, Riggs S, Fred HL. Bloody ascites: Diagnostic implications. *Am J Gastroenterol* 1969; 52:523–27.

[15]Harrison GN, Chew WH Jr. Tuberculous peritonitis. *South Med J* 1979; 72:1561–63.

[16]Judd DR, Starkloff GB, Zacharewicz FA. Tuberculous peritonitis. *South Med J* 1968; 61:797–800.

[17]Wolfe JHN, Behn AR, Jackson BT. Tuberculous peritonitis and the role of diagnostic laparoscopy. *Lancet* 1979; 1:852–53.

[18]Khoury GA, Payne CR, Harvey DR. Tuberculosis of the peritoneal cavity. *Br J Surg* 1978; 65:808–11.

[19]Sampliner RE, Iber FL. High protein ascites in patients with uncomplicated hepatic cirrhosis. *Am J Med Sci* 1974; 267:275–79.

[20]Rocco VK, Ware AJ. Cirrhotic ascites: Pathophysiology, diagnosis, and management. *Ann Intern Med* 1986; 105:573–85.

[21]Hoefs JC. The mechanism of ascitic fluid protein concentration increase during diuresis in patients with chronic liver disease. *Am J Gastroenterol* 1981; 76:423–31.

[22]Boyer TD, Kahn AM, Reynolds TB. Diagnostic value of ascitic fluid lactic dehydrogenase, protein, and WBC levels. *Arch Intern Med* 1978; 138:1103–1105.

[23]Garrison RN, Kaelin LD, Heuser LS, Galloway RH. Malignant ascites: Clinical and experimental observations. *Ann Surg* 1986; 203:644–51.

[24]Runyon BA, Hoefs JC, Morgan TR. Ascitic fluid analysis in malignancy-related ascites. *Hepatology* 1988; 8:1104–1109.

[25]Rovelstad RA, Bartholomew LG, Cain JC. Helpful laboratory procedures in the differential diagnosis of ascites. *Proc Mayo Clinic* 1959; 34:565–68.

[26]Sears D, Hajdu SI. The cytologic diagnosis of malignant neoplasms in pleural and peritoneal effusions. *Acta Cytol* 1987; 31(2):85–97.

[27]Gonnella JS, Hudson EK. Clinical patterns of tuberculous peritonitis. *Arch Intern Med* 1966; 117:164–69.

RED OR COLD DIARRHEA:
LESSONS FROM HISTORY*

Red-colored bowel movements can terrify the patient and sometimes mystify the doctor. The terror comes from fearing blood. The mystery comes when there is no blood. In virtually all such cases, a careful review of the patient's dietary and medication history will disclose the coloring agent. Foods known to be responsible are beets,[1] red peppers,[1] tomatoes,[2] red cherries,[3] "red hots,"[3] and breakfast cereal.[4] Oral medications that deserve consideration include the urinary analgesic phenazopyridine hydrochloride (Pyridium®),[5] the anthelmintic pyrvinium pamoate (Povan®),[1, 5] diazepam (Valium®) syrup,[6] and rifampin (Rifadin®).[7] Intravenous administration of sulfobromophthalein sodium (B.S.P.) to test liver function can also produce bloody-looking stools.[8]

Accounting for the red color doesn't necessarily end the story. In fact, paying attention to the *timing* of the stools in relation to intake of the coloring agent can be a shortcut to a short circuit. A recent report[9] described a woman who complained of watery diarrhea of ten days' duration. The diarrhea occurred shortly after each meal or after drinking fluids. It was generally unremarkable in appearance, but when the patient ate red gelatin, her stools became red within an

*Reprinted by permission from *Houston Medicine* 1990; 6:90.

hour. Persistent symptoms and continued weight loss prompted a barium enema examination, which demonstrated a gastrocolic fistula. Another patient with gastrocolic fistula experienced "cold" diarrhea approximately *five minutes* after drinking iced tea.[10]

The information presented here reminds us once again that a thoughtfully obtained and critically interpreted medical history is the cornerstone of diagnosis. Given the way medicine is being practiced these days, we need that reminder.

REFERENCES

[1]Seckler SG. Colorful pearls: Body excretions—feces. *Hospital Physician* 1979; December:52.

[2]Wiener SL, Wiener J. Red fruits causing false-positive occult blood tests in stool (*Letter*). *N Engl J Med* 1975; 293:408.

[3]Fred HL. Unreported observation.

[4]Payne JV. Benign red pigmentation of stool resulting from food coloring in a new breakfast cereal (the Franken Berry stool). *Pediatrics* 1972; 49:293–94.

[5]Drugs which may cause discoloration of the feces. *Hospital Formulary Management* 1975; February:64.

[6]Cotterill JA. Pink stools and diazepam syrup (*Letter*). *Lancet* 1974; 1:1062.

[7]*Physicians' Desk Reference.* 1989; 43:1420.

[8]Earnest JB, Fred HL, Eiband JM. Guaiac-negative "bloody" stool. *Br Med J* 1966; 2:703.

[9]Russell LJ, Kearl GW. Gastrocolic fistula presenting as acute diarrhea. *Am Fam Physician* 1989; October:223–25.

[10]McDaniel NT Jr, Bluth EI, Ray JE. Gastrocolic fistula in Crohn's disease. *Am J Gastroenterol* 1982; 77:588–89.

THE SCOPE OF SCOPES*

More than a century ago, Jean Martin Charcot[1] said: "We
see only what we are ready to see, what we have been taught
to see." Years later, Maxwell Wintrobe[2] wrote, "Many look, but
few see." These great physicians were emphasizing the same
thing: the power of observation. In Charcot's time, and to a
lesser extent during Wintrobe's career, skilled observation
was crucial because other diagnostic aids were limited. Today,
despite our advanced technology, we still need to *see* when we
look, as the following story exemplifies.

A thirty-year-old man complained of recurrent vomiting,
extreme polydipsia (35 to 50 glasses of water per day), and
progressive weight loss of four months' duration.
Hospitalization elsewhere had yielded no diagnosis. On
physical examination at our hospital, the only abnormality
noted was conspicuous weight loss. His peculiar constellation
of complaints coupled with the nonspecific physical findings
led to numerous consultations and a gamut of laboratory
investigations. Ultimately, tests showed hyperthyroidism.

When a colleague told me this story, I could understand
why the physicians involved didn't initially consider
hyperthyroidism. Recurrent vomiting as a manifestation of

*Reprinted by permission from the *Southern Medical Journal* 1990; 83:1205.

that illness is rare[3] and extreme polydipsia, virtually unheard of. Nevertheless, knowing that the patient was thyrotoxic, I suspected that at admission he had shown some physical evidence besides weight loss to suggest the diagnosis. So I asked his physician if we could examine him together.

I first saw the patient two weeks after he had received radioactive iodine therapy. His vomiting and polydipsia had diminished substantially. But his physician and I agreed that he had a prominent stare, distinct asymmetric exophthalmos, and subtle diffuse enlargement of the thyroid gland.

Doctors nowadays rely heavily on instruments other than their eyes and brains to help them see what they look at. One such instrument is "the scope," of which there are many:

angioscope	gonioscope
anoscope	laparoscope
bronchoscope	laryngoscope
choledochoscope	microscope
colonoscope	nasoscope
colposcope	ophthalmoscope
culdoscope	otoscope
cystoscope	peritoneoscope
duodenoscope	pharyngoscope
esophagoscope	sigmoidoscope
fluoroscope	thoracoscope
gastroscope	urethroscope

Of the scopes currently available, the oldest and most reliable is the retrospectoscope. As the case described illustrates, the retrospectoscope always gives a clear and meaningful view. It is our best teaching instrument.

Much more difficult to master than the retrospectoscope is the prospectoscope. Clarity and correctness of vision through *this* instrument are directly proportional to the competence of the user.

Once we are proficient in using both the retrospectoscope and the prospectoscope, we are ready to use the perspectoscope—the scope that all patients deserve. This scope brings everything into perspective and keeps it there.

REFERENCES

[1]Charcot JM (1825–1893), quoted by Strauss MB (Ed). *Familiar Medical Quotations.* Boston, Little, Brown and Co., 1968, p. 335.

[2]Wintrobe MM. *Blood, Pure and Eloquent.* New York, McGraw-Hill Book Co, 1980, p. 720.

[3]Rosenthal FD, Jones C, Lewis SI. Thyrotoxic vomiting. *Br Med J* 1976; 2:209–11.

THE CPC:
HISTORICAL CONSIDERATIONS, BENEFITS, AND DRAWBACKS*

Case Presentation

A forty-four-year-old black man was admitted to Hermann Hospital with chest pain, pretibial edema, and an erythematous scaly rash on his legs. The patient had experienced chest pain for the first time on the day of admission. It began while he was at rest following a day in which he lifted heavy boxes. The pain was right-sided, with a dull, tight, pressurelike quality; it did not radiate and was not pleuritic. He had no shortness of breath, nausea, vomiting, or diaphoresis. The pain resolved spontaneously within two hours, just as he arrived at the hospital.

Four months before admission he had been treated for a sore throat, sinus congestion, and a sore, red eye. Antibiotics, antihistamines, and decongestants gave no immediate relief. The eye continued to be swollen, and he was told he had

*Adapted from a clinicopathologic conference given by the author and others at the University of Texas Medical School at Houston on June 4, 1990. The full text of this conference appears elsewhere (Clinicopathologic Conference: A Black Man with Simultaneous Multisystem Disease. *Houston Medicine* 1990; 6:161–72).—ED.

conjunctivitis. He said that since then he has had temperatures to 102 F almost every day, a thirty-pound weight loss (despite increased appetite), and a sensation of burning on the bottom of his feet.

Within the previous two months, he had developed swelling of his feet and calves and had noted a severe irritating dryness of the skin on his legs. He reported no orthopnea, dyspnea on exertion, or paroxysmal nocturnal dyspnea. On the day of admission, the left side of his face felt weak and his left eyelid drooped slightly.

TABLE 1: LABORATORY VALUES UPON ADMISSION

Serum values:

White blood cell count ..... 7,300/cu mm
Polymorphonuclears 39%
Band neutrophils 8%
Lymphocytes 17%
Monocytes 20%
Eosinophils 16%
Hemoglobin .... 11.8 gm/dL
Hematocrit 36%
Mean corpuscular volume ...... 79/cu μg
Prothrombin time .... 12.4 sec.
(normal: ⟨ 13.1)
Partial thromboplastin time ... 26.2 sec.
(normal: ⟨ 35)

Electrolytes:
Sodium .... 133 mmol/L
Potassium .... 3.6 mmol/L
Chloride .... 97 mmol/L
Carbon dioxide .... 26 mmol/L
Glucose .... 94 mg/dL
Creatinine .... 2.6 mg/dL
Urea nitrogen .... 25 mg/dL
Total protein .... 9 g/dL
Albumin .... 2.9 g/dL
Calcium .... 10.1 mg/dL
Phosphorus .... 4.3 mg/dL

Uric acid .... 6.5 mg/dL
SGOT .... 87 U/L (normal: ⟨ 40)
SGPT .... 103 U/L (normal: ⟨ 40)
Alkaline phosphatase .... 180 U/L
(normal: 30–130)
Lactate dehydrogenase .... 381 U/L
(normal: 100–225)
Total bilirubin .... 0.8 mg/dL
Cholesterol .... 210 mg/dL
Triglycerides .... 169 mg/dL
Sedimentation rate .... 49 mm/hr
(norm: 0–10)
HIV titer .... neg.
Creatine kinase .... 934 and 693 U/L
MB fractions .... ⟨ 2.5%

Urine values:
Specific gravity 1.025
Protein .... 1+
Glucose .... neg.
Ketones .... neg.
White blood cells 3–5
Red blood cells 2–4
Protein 1.3 gm/24-hr
(normal: 0–0.8 g)

Skin test: .... anergic

The patient had been healthy until the onset of these symptoms. He gave no history of cough, blood in his urine, diarrhea, diabetes, hypertension, or elevated cholesterol level. He had not traveled recently, had no recent insect bites, andhad never used intravenous or illicit drugs, alcohol, or tobacco. His only medication before this admission was ibuprofen for generalized aches. His father had a myocardial infarction at the age of 65 years.

Physical examination

At admission, the patient was alert, in no respiratory distress, and appeared healthy. His temperature was 99 F, pulse rate was 80 beats per minute, respirations were 16 per minute, and blood pressure was 172/92 mm Hg without orthostatic change.

The skin of the lower legs demonstrated severe scaling; large dry scales adhered to the skin. No petechiae, bruising, or lymphadenopathy was noted. There was 3 + pitting edema over the pretibial areas. There was no penetrating wound of the skin. No Homan's sign was present. The extremities showed no clubbing, cyanosis, or splinter hemorrhages.

Facial asymmetry was present, with a left seventh cranial nerve deficit and flattening of the nasolabial fold. The parotid glands were mildly enlarged. The left eye was erythematous, with small yellow nodules on the conjunctiva. The pupils were 4 mm and normally reactive. There was no scleral icterus. On funduscopic examination, no exudates or hemorrhages were seen; the discs were flat. The tongue and tonsils were mildly erythematous.

Auscultation of the lungs demonstrated bilateral basilar crackles. The heart had a regular rate and rhythm with normal first and second heart sounds. A fourth heart sound was present, and there was a grade II/IV systolic murmur at the left sternal border. No gallop or rub was heard. No pulsus paradoxus was present.

On abdominal examination, bowel sounds were normal; there was no protuberance or fluid wave. The liver span was 10 cm; the tip of the spleen was not felt. Rectal examination showed no masses. The stool was negative for occult blood.

The only evidence of muscle weakness was the seventh cranial nerve deficit. Sensory and gait examinations were normal. No nystagmus was present.

Laboratory data

Serum and urine values and results of a skin test are given in Table 1.

The chest roentgenograms were interpreted as showing bilateral hilar adenopathy with reticulonodular disease prominent in the bases. The possibility of small pleural effusions could not be ruled out. No decubitus films were made.

The electrocardiograms showed nonspecific ST-T wave changes. The voltage was increased over the precordium, which could indicate left ventricular enlargement. There was evidence of left atrial enlargement.

A diagnostic procedure was performed.

Clinical Discussion

Herbert L. Fred, M.D., Professor, Department
of Internal Medicine
The University of Texas Medical School at Houston

Because my discussion of today's case will be relatively brief, I'll take a few minutes to comment on CPCs in general. I've been associated with CPCs for exactly forty years— initially as an attendee, then as an abstractor or discussant, and always as an interested reader. Based on that experience, I regard the CPC as an excellent educational exercise. From it, physicians can learn not only factual information but also the value of a well-organized, step-by-step approach to clinical problem solving. Yet CPCs also have some *negative* aspects that I will mention as I go along. But first, some historical perspective.

CPCs originated in Boston in 1900. They began as informal discussions in the private office of Dr. Richard C. Cabot, a prominent Harvard internist. Cabot had gotten the idea for this case method of teaching medicine from Walter B. Cannon, who was a medical student at Harvard. Cannon, in turn, had gotten the idea from his roommate, who was a law student.

Ultimately, the CPCs moved from Cabot's office to the
Massachusetts General Hospital, where they were called the
Cabot Clinicopathologic Conferences. In 1924, *The Boston
Medical and Surgical Journal* started publishing these
conferences. Four years later, that journal became *The New
England Journal of Medicine,* wherein CPCs have been a
feature ever since.

At Johns Hopkins Hospital, CPCs were the highlight of my
medical school training. Every Wednesday at noon, we
crammed into a dimly lit, smoke-filled room to hear the
chairman of medicine, Dr. A. McGehee Harvey, match wits
with the chairman of pathology, Dr. Arnold Rich. Both were
giants in their respective fields, and both, with rare
exceptions, conducted the CPC *every week.* The opportunity
to observe their analytical minds in action on a regular basis
for four straight years was a unique and unforgettable
privilege.

In those days at Hopkins, the clinician wasn't asked to base
his discussion on a clinical abstract prepared by a third party.
He prepared the abstract himself. The complete clinical
record in its original state was available to him. He had the
raw notes of the students, the house officers, the nurses, the
attending physicians, and everyone else who contributed to
the record. This gave him a better appreciation of the total
situation that existed during the patient's hospital stay. His
abstract usually was about a page and a half in length and
concentrated on the patient's medical history and physical
findings.

Nowadays, the protocol is prepared by a "third party," is
often many pages long, and typically emphasizes laboratory
data. (The protocol for today's case is a pleasant exception to
that trend.) By moving from the bedside to the laboratory, we
are becoming proficient in ordering tests, but deficient in
taking a pertinent medical history and doing a good physical
examination. As a clinician and as a patient, I find that trade-
off uneven and unfortunate.

Under the rules of a CPC, the discussant cannot question
or examine the patient personally. Nor can he obtain
additional laboratory studies that he might want. He must
work instead with what is given him, which means that he

must view the patient through the eyes and brains of others. Fortunately, such rules don't apply to the actual practice of medicine. A good doctor always talks with and examines the patient himself, trusting himself—not others—to make the diagnosis. Shakespeare underscored that principle when he wrote, "Let every eye negotiate for itself and trust no agent."[1]

The discussant in a CPC typically spends hours—sometimes days or weeks—preparing his remarks, and his presentation ordinarily follows a standard format. He begins his analysis by selecting the most important or dominant feature of the patient's illness. Next, he reviews in detail the various causes of that feature, systematically eliminating all but the one he believes best explains most or all of the findings in the case.

That approach to clinical problem solving is ideal, but it isn't always practical or necessary. In the real world, few if any physicians can devote hours or days to every diagnostic challenge they face. Their work load is too great. Thus, many of them turn to a gamut of tests and myriad consultants for help. Others—the more seasoned clinicians—rely heavily on pattern recognition. Diseases, like people, have their own characteristics. And like people, certain diseases bear striking resemblances to one another. But differentiation is nearly always possible if we know what to look for and how to find it.

TABLE 2: CAUSES OF WIDESPREAD MULTISYSTEM DISEASE

1) Widespread malignant neoplasm

2) Infiltrative process
    Sarcoidosis
    Hemachromatosis
    Amyloidosis, etc.

3) Disseminated infection
    Mycobacterial   Protozoal
    Viral   Fungal
    Spirochetal   Bacterial

4) Circulatory disturbance
    Peripheral—
        primary vasculitis
        connective tissue disorder
        embolic
    Central—
        cardiac

One more point deserves attention. Many physicians figure that CPCs involve some sort of trickery. As a consequence, they assume that the case in question is not diagnosable clinically, is not what it appears to be, is a rare disease, or is an entity only recently reported. I don't subscribe to such preconceptions because they thwart open-mindedness and blunt our ability to see things as they are. Furthermore, selecting a case to trick rather than to test the discussant defeats the purpose of the CPC. So much for the negative aspects of these exercises.

Now for today's case. In line with tradition, I could pick hilar adenopathy, a scaly rash, parotid enlargement, hyperglobulinemia, or a facial palsy as possible starting points for discussion. The truly dominant feature of this case, however, is simultaneous multisystem disease in a healthy-appearing man. Causes of simultaneous multisystem disease are listed in Table 2. Our patient clearly had one of those disorders.

The initial protocol I received didn't mention a chest film or an electrocardiogram. So I formulated my diagnosis from the patient's history and physical examination—a principle of good medicine being uprooted by the gimmicks and gadgets that pervade our profession. When the chest films became available, they put icing on the diagnostic cake I had already baked.

Another principle of good medicine applies to this case: Knowing that you *know* is just as important as knowing that you *don't* know. For example, if you see an animal that has webbed feet and feathers, lives in and around water, and goes "quack-quack," you *know* it's a duck. And you don't have to rely on tests and consultants to rule out a chicken, a fish, or a rabbit. Similarly, when you see a black patient who reports a thirty-pound weight loss and four months of fever; who demonstrates a facial palsy, an inflamed eye with nodules in the conjunctiva, bilateral parotid enlargement, an erythematous scaly rash, and bilateral hilar adenopathy with reticulo-nodular lung disease; and who, despite all of these abnormalities, appears healthy—you know he has *sarcoidosis.* Nothing else fits.

Primary diagnoses other than sarcoidosis did come to mind in this case—but only fleetingly. They were granulomatous infection, particularly tuberculosis and fungal disease; lymphomas of all types, including the Sézary mycosis fungoides complex; lymphomatoid granulomatosis; vasculitis; and connective tissue disorders. I found little, however, to support these or any other possibilities, either as primary diagnoses or as diseases coexisting with or masquerading as sarcoidosis.[2-6]

Sarcoidosis explains not only our patient's facial palsy,[7] inflamed eye,[8, 9] parotid enlargement,[10, 11] and erythematous scaly rash,[12, 13] but also his history of fever[14] and weight loss[12, 15] as well as his lymphopenia,[16] eosinophilia,[17] monocytosis,[17] anergy,[18] serum enzyme derangements,[19-21] urinary changes,[22, 23] and hyperglobulinemia.[24, 25] His bilateral hilar adenopathy[26, 27] and reticulo-nodular lung disease[28, 29] are classic for sarcoidosis, too.

That ends the easy part of this case. The hard part is explaining the chest pain that prompted the patient's admission, the densities that subsequently appeared in his costophrenic areas, and the pre-existing pitting edema of his lower extremities. I don't know what caused his chest pain, but I suspect it was unrelated to sarcoidosis. The type of pain and the elevated plasma creatine kinase levels suggest coronary artery disease with possible myocardial infarction. But the location of the pain was not typical for coronary artery disease, the electrocardiographic changes were nonspecific, and the MB fraction accounted for less than 2.5% of the total creatine kinase activity.[30] Furthermore, many noncardiac conditions such as lung disease,[31, 32] muscle disease[32] (including sarcoid myopathy[19, 20]), and even the intramuscular injection of various medications[33, 34] can cause substantial increases in plasma concentrations of creatine kinase. These arguments aside, if the disease process in the costophrenic areas represented early bilateral effusions—and I think it did—the preceding chest pain would favor an acute cardiac

insult with new onset heart failure or worsening of already
established heart failure. Though cardiac sarcoidosis can
certainly cause heart failure, it more commonly produces
arrhythmia, heart block, or sudden death.[35]

Could the disease process in the costophrenic areas be
pulmonary infection, infarction, neoplasm, or atelectasis?
Those possibilities always deserve consideration when
unexplained densities appear on chest film, but the evidence
we have suggests otherwise. The pain, for example, was not
pleuritic and was on the right side, while the acute basilar
changes were more prominent on the left side. In addition, the
patient appeared healthy and had no fever or respiratory
complaints at admission.

Concerning the $3+$ pitting edema, the protocol doesn't say
how far up the legs the fluid extended. It does say, however,
that for two months the patient had noted swelling of his
calves as well as his feet. I will assume that his calves swelled
from surrounding fluid rather than from sarcoid myopathy.[20]

In my experience as a general internist, the most common
cause of chronic, symmetrical swelling of the feet and lower
legs has been heart failure. Against that diagnosis in this
patient—but not excluding it—are the absence of any
weakness or exertional dyspnea, the normal heart size on
chest film, and no evident pulmonary vascular congestion. Yet
in the face of parenchymal lung disease, pulmonary vascular
congestion can be difficult to detect. Moreover, engorged main
pulmonary arteries can be mistaken for bilateral hilar
adenopathy.[26] The inspiratory effort on the second chest film
was comparatively reduced. This could magnify the acute
basilar changes, but it couldn't explain them entirely. If one
accepts the premise that small pleural effusions developed
rapidly in this patient, a failing heart would be the prime
suspect. The cause of such heart failure, however, would be
conjectural at best.

The patient's serum albumin level of 2.9 gm/100 ml was not
low enough to induce edema, and there is little to support
venous thromboses as the cause of the symmetrical swelling.
At least two patients with sarcoidosis have had massive *lymph
edema* of the lower extremities associated with sarcoid
involvement of the retroperitoneal[36] and inguinal[37] lymph
nodes, respectively. Consequently, blockage of lymph flow

conceivably could have been operative in our patient. Or
perhaps the edema resulted from capillary leakage related to
the skin disease of his legs. All things considered, I don't have
enough data to decide with confidence which, if any, of these
mechanisms—singularly or in concert—accounted for the
fluid accumulation in this patient.

The diagnostic procedure referred to in the protocol
should have been a biopsy. I would have biopsied the
conjunctival nodules[38] or the skin lesions first, chiefly because
of the relative ease and safety of such an approach. If those
biopsies had proved negative or inconclusive, I would have
biopsied his bronchial mucosa, a common site for sarcoid
granulomata in patients with mediastinal or pulmonary
sarcoidosis.[39, 40] Transbronchial lung biopsy, open-lung biopsy,
and mediastinoscopy would be other options to consider in
today's case. I don't believe biopsy of the bone marrow[41] or
liver[21] would have helped.

Some physicians accept the diagnosis of sarcoidosis
without biopsy confirmation when bilateral hilar adenopathy
occurs in asymptomatic patients with normal physical
examinations or in patients with erythema nodosum or
uveitis.[27] Others accept the diagnosis if the clinical picture is
suggestive and biopsy at one or more sites shows
noncaseating granulomata.[8, 9] Still others believe that the
diagnosis should remain suspect until extensive and
continued search fails to uncover any infectious agent or
neoplasm capable of producing clinicopathologic findings
similar to those of sarcoidosis.[2, 42, 43] In my opinion, the extent
and duration of such studies should be tailored to the
individual patient and will depend largely on the physician's
medical knowledge and clinical experience.

To summarize:

1) When you see a healthy-appearing black patient with a
facial palsy, think of sarcoidosis, and get a chest film. If the
chest film shows bilateral hilar adenopathy, sarcoidosis is
virtually certain. In fact, bilateral hilar adenopathy, by itself,

should bring to mind sarcoidosis, lymphoma, and metastatic carcinoma—in that order.[26, 27]

2) If the patient has facial palsy, bilateral hilar adenopathy, and inflammation of one or both eyes, the inflammation likely represents sarcoid uveitis or conjunctivitis.

3) If the patient has inflammation of one or both eyes and also has parotid enlargement and fever, think of uveo-parotid fever, a syndrome characteristic of sarcoidosis.[44] Facial palsy often accompanies that syndrome.

4) If the patient has facial palsy, bilateral hilar adenopathy, inflammation of one or both eyes, parotid enlargement, and an erythematous scaly rash, the rash probably represents sarcoidosis, too.

Finally this:

A CPC that I attended as a medical student involved a particularly complex case. The discussant was Dr. Charles Baker, a visiting professor from Guy's Hospital in London. His presentation was awe-inspiring, and I'll never forget his concluding remark: "Therefore, ladies and gentlemen, this patient could *only* have primary amyloidosis." He was right.

My discussion today pales in comparison with the one he gave, but I will conclude with a remark similar to the one he made: "Therefore, ladies and gentlemen, this patient's primary disease could *only* be multisystem sarcoidosis."

Pathologic Findings and Clinical Follow-Up

A biopsy of the scaly rash showed noncaseating granulomas in the dermis, consistent with sarcoidosis. The patient received steroid therapy and was discharged from the hospital. At follow-up examination, his skin lesions and inflamed eye had improved considerably. The exact cause of his pretibial edema and costophrenic densities was not determined.

REFERENCES

[1]Shakespeare. *Much Ado about Nothing*, 2.1.184.

[2]Sicherman HJ, Andersen HA, DeRemee RA. Sarcoidosis or fungal disease? *Chest* 1973; 64:36–38.

[3]Goldfarb BL, Cohen SS. Coexistent disseminated sarcoidosis and Hodgkin's disease. *JAMA* 1970; 211:1525–28.

[4]Spitzer T, Crum E, Schacter L, Abboud S. Case report: Sarcoidosis, Hodgkin's disease, and autoimmune hemolytic anemia. *Am J Med Sci* 1986; 291:190–93.

[5]Winterbauer RH, Kraemer KG. The infectious complications of sarcoidosis. A current perspective. *Arch Intern Med* 1976; 136:1356–62.

[6]James DG. Sarcoidosis. In *Disease-a-Month.* Chicago, Year Book Publishers, Inc., 1970, p. 9.

[7]Stern BJ, Krumholz A, Johns C, *et al.* Sarcoidosis and its neurological manifestations. *Arch Neurol* 1985; 42:909–17.

[8]Obenauf CD, Shaw HE, Sydnor CF, Klintworth GK. Sarcoidosis and its ophthalmic manifestations. *Am J Ophthalmol* 1978; 86:648–55.

[9]Karma A, Huhti E, Poukkula A. Course and outcome of ocular sarcoidosis. *Am J Ophthalmol* 1988; 106:467–72.

[10]Greenberg G, Anderson R, Sharpstone P, James DG. Enlargement of parotid gland due to sarcoidosis. *Br Med J* 1964; 2:861–62.

[11]Iko BO, Chinwuba CE, Myers EM, Teal JS. Sarcoidosis of the parotid gland. *Br J Radiol* 1986; 59:547–52.

[12]Mora RG, Gullung WH. Sarcoidosis: A case with unusual manifestations. *South Med J* 1980; 73:1063–65.

[13]Kauh YC, Goody HE, Luscombe HA. Ichthyosiform sarcoidosis. *Arch Dermatol* 1978; 114:100-101.

[14]Nolan JP, Klatskin G. The fever of sarcoidosis. *Ann Intern Med* 1964; 61:455–61.

[15]Longcope WT, Freiman DG. *A Study of Sarcoidosis.* Baltimore, The Williams & Wilkins Company, 1952, p. 35.

[16]Hoffbrand BI. Occurrence and significance of lymphopenia in sarcoidosis. *Am Rev Respir Dis* 1968; 98:107–10.

[17]Wintrobe MM, Lee GR, Boggs DR, *et al. Clinical Hematology.* Philadelphia, Lea & Febiger, 1974, pp. 1283, 1287.

[18]Daniele RP, Dauber JH, Rossman MD. Immunologic abnormalities in sarcoidosis. *Ann Intern Med* 1980; 92:406–16.

[19]Ando DG, Lynch JP III, Fantone JC III. Sarcoid myopathy with elevated creatine phosphokinase. *Am Rev Respir Dis* 1985; 131:298–300.

[20]Matteson EL, Michet CJ. Sarcoid myositis with pseudohypertrophy. *Am J Med* 1989; 87:240–41.

[21]Israel HL, Margolis ML, Rose LJ. Hepatic granulomatosis and sarcoidosis. Further observations. *Dig Dis Sci* 1984; 29:353–56.

[22]Romer FK. Renal manifestations and abnormal calcium metabolism in sarcoidosis. *Quart J Med* 1980; 49:233–47.

[23]Muther RS, McCarron DA, Bennett WM. Renal manifestations of sarcoidosis. *Arch Intern Med* 1981; 141:643–45.

[24]Greenberg G, Feizi T, James DG, Bird R. Serum-proteins in sarcoidosis. *Lancet* 1964; 2:1313–15.

[25]Goldstein RA, Israel HL. An assessment of serum protein electrophoresis in sarcoidosis. *Am J Med Sci* 1968; 256:306–13.

[26]Hodgson CH, Olsen AM, Good CA. Bilateral hilar adenopathy: Its significance and management. *Ann Intern Med* 1955; 43:83–99.

[27]Winterbauer RH, Belic N, Moores KD. A clinical interpretation of bilateral hilar adenopathy. *Ann Intern Med* 1973; 78:65–71.

[28]Kirks DR, McCormick VD, Greenspan RH. Pulmonary sarcoidosis. Roentgenologic analysis of 150 patients. *Am J Roentgenol Rad Ther Nucl Med* 1973; 117:777–86.

[29]Reisner D. Observations on the course and prognosis of sarcoidosis. With special considerations of its intrathoracic manifestations. *Am Rev Respir Dis* 1967; 96:361–80.

[30]Roberts R. Where, oh where has the MB gone? *N Engl J Med* 1985; 313:1081–83.

[31]Perkoff GT. Demonstration of creatine phosphokinase in human lung tissue. *Arch Intern Med* 1968; 122:326–28.

[32]Nevins MA, Saran M, Bright M, Lyon LJ. Pitfalls in interpreting serum creatine phosphokinase activity. *JAMA* 1973; 224:1382–87.

[33]Cacace L. Elevated serum CPK after drug injections. *N Engl J Med* 1972; 287:309–10.

[34]Rose S, Price PG. Effect of intramuscular injections on serum creatine phosphokinase. *JAMA* 1973; 225:417.

[35]Roberts WC, McAllister HA Jr, Ferrans VJ. Sarcoidosis of the heart. A clinicopathologic study of 35 necropsy patients (group I) and review of 78 previously described necropsy patients (group II). *Am J Med* 1977; 63:86–108.

[36]Silver HM, Tsangaris NT, Eaton OM. Lymphedema and lymphography in sarcoidosis. *Arch Intern Med* 1966; 117:712–14.

[37]Nathan MPR, Pinsker R, Chase PH, Elguezabel A. Sarcoidosis presenting as lymphedema. *Arch Dermatol* 1974; 109:543–44.

[38]Karcioglu ZA, Brear R. Conjunctival biopsy in sarcoidosis. *Am J Ophthalmol* 1985; 99:68–73.

[39]Mitchell DM, Mitchell DN, Collins JV, Emerson CJ. Transbronchial lung biopsy through fibreoptic bronchoscope in diagnosis of sarcoidosis. *Br Med J* 1980; 280:679–81.

[40]Armstrong JR, Radke JR, Kvale PA, *et al.* Endoscopic findings in sarcoidosis. Characteristics and correlations with radiographic staging and bronchial mucosal biopsy yield. *Ann Otol* 1981; 90:339–43.

[41]Ellman L. Bone marrow biopsy in the evaluation of lymphoma, carcinoma and granulomatous disorders. *Am J Med* 1976; 60:1–7.

[42]Baum GL, Schwarz J, Barlow PB. Sarcoidosis and specific etiologic agents: A continuing enigma. *Chest* 1973; 63:488–94.

[43]James DG. Sarcoidosis. In *Disease-a-Month.* Chicago, Year Book Medical Publishers, Inc., 1970, pp. 25–26.

[44]Longcope WI, Freiman DG. *A Study of Sarcoidosis.* Baltimore: The Williams and Wilkins Company, 1952, pp. 88–92.

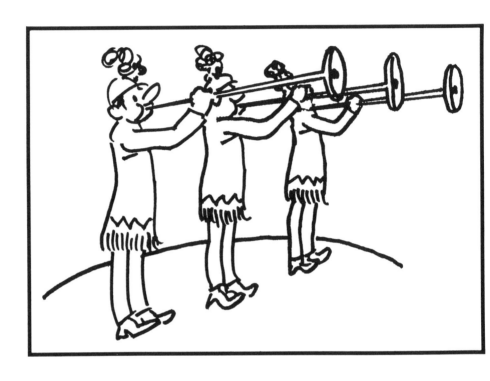

FOR MENTORS ONLY

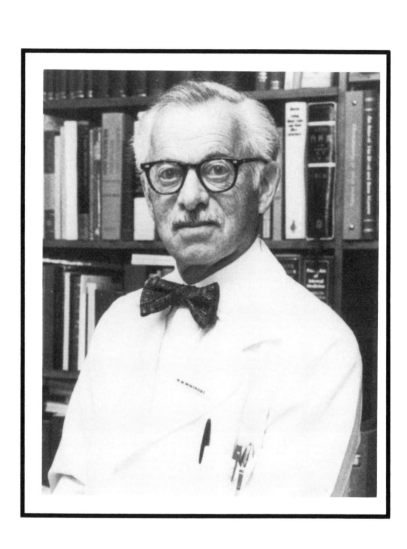

A GREAT LEADER*

Someone once said, "A good leader inspires men to have confidence in him; a great leader inspires them to have confidence in themselves."† In that light and in a host of other ways, Maxwell Myer Wintrobe, M.D., Ph.D.—perhaps the world's foremost hematologist—was, indeed, a great leader. His death on December 9, 1986, at the age of eighty-five, ended six decades of outstanding clinical research and teaching.

Dr. Wintrobe was born October 27, 1901 in Halifax, Nova Scotia, Canada. He earned his degree in Medicine from the University of Manitoba in 1926 and a Ph.D. from Tulane University in 1929. The following year he joined the faculty of Johns Hopkins University and eventually became Physician-in-Charge, Clinic for Nutritional, Gastro-Intestinal, and Hemopoietic Disorders at the Johns Hopkins Hospital.

He left Baltimore in 1943 and went to the University of Utah as its first professor and head of the Department of Internal Medicine. Upon arriving in Salt Lake City, he found the medical school housed in a World War I dormitory for cavalry officers. Undaunted, he strove tirelessly to help the School of

*Reprinted by permission from *Houston Medical Journal* 1987; 3:3–4.

†From McKenzie EC (Ed.). *14,000 Quips & Quotes for Writers and Speakers.* New York, Greenwich House, 1984, p. 221.

Medicine achieve the international recognition it now enjoys. He was instrumental in getting the school its first research grant—$100,000 to study muscular dystrophy and other hereditary and metabolic disorders. It was the first research grant ever awarded by the National Institutes of Health. He chaired the Department of Internal Medicine until 1967; in 1970 he was named Distinguished Professor of Internal Medicine, the university's highest academic rank.

Dr. Wintrobe's interest in hematology began when he was a medical student working part-time in the hospital's blood bank. This job ignited a curiosity that culminated in his countless contributions to our understanding of the blood and its diseases. He devised the red blood cell indices—MCV (mean corpuscular volume), MCH (mean corpuscular hemoglobin), and MCHC (mean corpuscular hemoglobin concentration). Based on these indices, he introduced a morphologic classification of anemias that is used everywhere. He developed an apparatus, the Wintrobe hematocrit, that reliably measures the volume of packed red blood cells; gave the first account of a cryoglobulin in the blood; offered the first description of Fabry's disease in an American patient; provided the first evidence that Cooley's anemia (thalassemia major) is a homozygous disorder; emphasized the role of nutritional factors, particularly the B vitamins, in hemopoiesis; and successfully produced pernicious anemia in swine. Additionally, he pioneered in studying the effects of nitrogen mustard, folate antagonists, and adrenocorticosteroids on the hemopoietic system; called attention to the potential of chloramphenicol to produce aplastic anemia; and led the drive to recognize and publicize adverse reactions to drugs.

He wrote 400 medical articles and three books. His text *Clinical Hematology* has been the standard in its field for forty-five years. His *Blood, Pure and Eloquent: A Story of Discovery, of People, and of Ideas* (McGraw-Hill Book Company, New York) won the yearly American Medical

Writers Association book award for physicians in 1980. His third book, *Hematology, the Blossoming of a Science: A Story of Inspiration and Effort* (Lea & Febiger, Philadelphia) was published two years ago. He was coeditor of *Harrison's Principles of Internal Medicine* from 1951 through 1966; was its editor-in-chief for the sixth and seventh editions in 1970 and 1974; and held editorial posts with twenty-two other publications.

Dr. Wintrobe lectured in numerous countries, received myriad awards for his research and teaching, headed many prestigious organizations and committees, and trained hundreds of house officers and scores of hematologists. In 1980, I wrote a tribute to him.‡ My thoughts then hold true today.

‡That tribute appears in my first book, *Elephant Medicine—And More: Musings of a Medical Educator.* Macon, Mercer University Press, 1988, pp. 23–25.

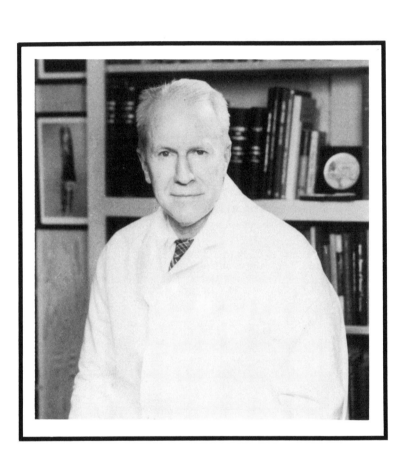

WILLIAM B. BEAN:
A TRIBUTE*

On March 1, 1989, cancer ended the glorious career of William B. Bean, M.D. As a consequence, the medical world lost one of its few remaining giants, and I lost a true friend.

Though known best for his work in nutrition, rare diseases, myocardial infarction, and the history of medicine, Bill was equally at home in the classroom, at the bedside, or in the laboratory. After obtaining his medical degree from the University of Virginia School of Medicine, he continued residency training at Johns Hopkins Hospital and Cincinnati General Hospital. For twenty-two years, from 1948 to 1970, he was professor and head of the Department of Internal Medicine at the University of Iowa College of Medicine. From 1974 to 1980, he was the director of the Institute for the Medical Humanities at the University of Texas Medical Branch in Galveston. In 1980 Bill returned to the University of Iowa College of Medicine to teach as the Sir William Osler Professor of Medicine.

His curriculum vitae totaled 200 typewritten pages and included 527 articles, 118 books or chapters in books, and 693 book reviews. He also presented more than 800 formal lectures. The breadth of his interests is evident from the following sampling of his many memberships, offices, and honors: first president, American Osler Society; fellow and governor,

*Reprinted by permission from *Houston Medicine* 1989; 5:43–45.

American College of Cardiology; president, Iowa Chapter,
Archeology Institute of America; consultant to the Surgeon
General, U.S. Army; fellow and vice president,
American Association for the Advancement of Science; fellow,
Royal Society of Medicine, London; president, American Clinical
and Climatological Association; member, American Association
of Medical History; charter member, American College of Sports
Medicine; and fellow, American Medical Writers Association.

Bill had exceptional editorial skills and experience. For five
years he was editor-in-chief of the *Archives of Internal Medicine*
and for fourteen years was editor of *Stedman's Medical
Dictionary.* He was a contributing editor to *Encyclopaedia
Britannica* and an associate editor or member of the editorial
boards of the *Journal of Clinical Investigation, Journal of
Laboratory and Clinical Medicine, Diseases of the Chest,
Medicine, Journal of Medical Education, American Journal of
Clinical Nutrition,* and many other distinguished publications.
Houston Medicine was honored to have him as a senior editorial
consultant.

When Bill learned that he had metastatic cancer, he wrote
the following letter to a colleague:

> Dear Jack:
>
> I thought I'd send for your information the current account of
> my state of health or lack of it, so I am enclosing the letter that I
> dispatched to my two sisters and brother and our three children
> after I got the pathology report of the bronchoscopic
> examination. I am still coming to work every day but choose my
> own hours. I am not sitting around idle waiting for the sword of
> Damocles to fall. It is interesting to have such a personal
> experience in Thanatopsis.
>
> Yr serv't,
Bill

The colleague then notified me and I, in turn, wrote a long
letter to Bill, part of which follows:

> Though I was never one of your students, I have always
> considered you as one of my teachers. You, more than anyone
> else, taught me the value of studying and reporting on "rare"
> diseases. You also instilled in me the desire to write well and
> convinced me of the need to communicate effectively. I often

refer to you and your work when I try to show medical students and house officers the right way to do things.

In summary, Bill, you have had a profoundly positive influence on my career. You have been my role model, my advisor, and my friend. And as I reflect on your current situation, two of your magnificent qualities stand out—courage and strength. You are an inspiration.

Yr Stud't,
Herb

A month later, Bill responded, in part:

I am a little dilatory in getting responses to the outpouring of letters that I got because Jack sent around the melancholy news to the members of the Osler Society. I think the letters I got from you and from Carlton Chapman rank highest in reminding me of the long trail of friendship that with you both had many peaks. . . .

He ended the letter with this:

I won't say that getting letters like yours is worth getting the illness, but it certainly is an inspiration to me, and I have not ever been impervious to flattery, though I don't think I've been swept off my feet by it. Again, I deeply appreciate your kindness and wisdom and especially your friendship.

Yr friend and serv't,
Bill

Logan Pearsall Smith once said, "There are two things to aim at in life: first to get what you want, and, after that, to enjoy it. Only the wisest of mankind achieve the second."

Bill Bean was, indeed, among the wisest of mankind.

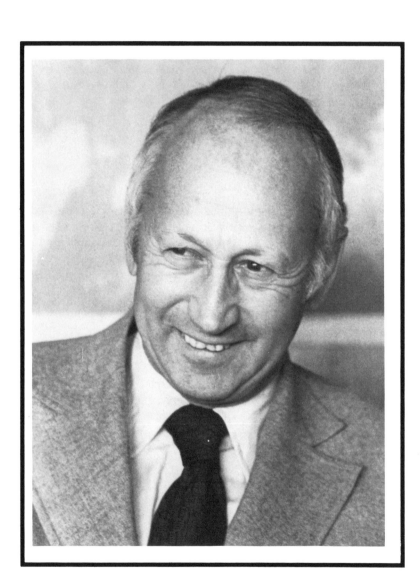

A REAL MENSCH*

When great people die, it is customary and appropriate to cite their contributions to humankind. In that light, I have used this column to memorialize my mentor Maxwell Wintrobe[1] and my friend William Bean,[2] both giants of medicine. Now I pay tribute to another giant whose mark on medicine and the world deserves our attention.

This person died suddenly on November 30, 1990, at the age of seventy-five. I had met him for the first and only time one month earlier during a luncheon meeting of the American Medical Writers Association. He was the featured speaker, and we sat at the same table. Contrary to my expectations, he was extraordinarily down to earth and exceptionally friendly. And his hour-long speech, delivered without notes, was the most captivating I have ever heard.

*Reprinted by permission from *Houston Medicine* 1991; 7:41.

He received many honors. He was adjunct professor in the School of Medicine at the University of California at Los Angeles. He held the only honorary degree in medicine awarded jointly by the Yale University School of Medicine, Connecticut Medical Association, and New Haven County Medical Society. He served on the Advisory Board of Harvard University's Center for Health Communication and of Duke University Medical School's Comprehensive Cancer Care Center. He was a trustee of the American Institute of Stress and of the Institute for the Advancement of Health. He earned the United Nations Peace Medal, the American Peace Award, and the Personal Medallion of Pope John XXIII. He also got the City of Hiroshima Award for carrying out medical rehabilitative projects for victims of the bombing there.

His accomplishments in the medical arena are all the more remarkable given that he was neither a physician nor a scientist. He was, instead, the celebrated editor of the *Saturday Review* for thirty-five years; the author of twenty-five books; and a diplomatic emissary for Presidents Eisenhower, Kennedy, and Johnson.

In Yiddish, *mensch* refers to a thoroughly admirable man. Norman Cousins was indeed a real mensch.

REFERENCES

[1]Fred HL. A great leader. *Houston Medical Journal* 1987; 3:3–5.

[2]Fred HL. William B. Bean: A tribute. *Houston Medicine* 1989; 5:43–45.

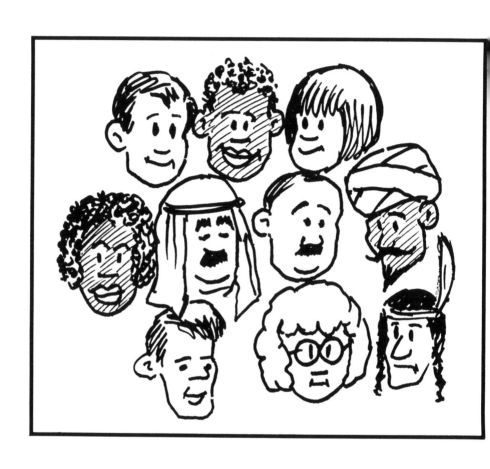

FOR EVERYBODY ONLY

Many careers reflect ascent by assent.

H.L.F.

—in "As a Matter of 'Fact'. . ."

FOUR-LETTER WORDS*

In today's world, "four-letter word" is an imprecise term with a precise connotation. Everybody knows that it's the nice way of referring to not-so-nice words. And just about everybody hears, sees, says, or thinks four-letter words daily.

But today's world would be better off if we spent less time broadcasting four-letter words and more time exchanging "four-word letters." After all, nobody doesn't like a "thank you very much."

*Reprinted by permission from the *Southern Medical Journal* 1990; 83:563.

AS A MATTER OF "FACT". . .*

Truth is one forever absolute, but opinion is truth filtered through the moods, the blood, the disposition of the spectator.
—*Wendell Phillips*
Idols, 1859

Fact:

The world is flat.

This "fact," once widely accepted, turned out to be an opinion.

Opinion:

The earth moves.

This "opinion," propounded by Aristarchus of Samos (c. 310–230 B.C. *) was, instead, a fact.*

How do we differentiate fact from opinion? Ordinarily, the question doesn't arise. Everyone knows that certain things are facts (the length of a mile, the outcome of World War II), while other things are opinions (best movie, smartest student, finest cigar). Yet, from time to time, we all present opinions as if they were facts.

When people render opinions as facts, they don't intend to mislead. But misunderstandings are inevitable. The difficulty

*Reprinted by permission from the *Southern Medical Journal* 1990; 83:203–204.

stems from the way we perceive what is said. Our perceptions, in turn, are the product of our childhood experiences, educational background, financial status, social position, and self-image. To complicate matters, we frequently hear only what we want to hear and see only what we look for. We also tend to regard as fact anything that agrees with our preconceived notions or that originates from someone we respect. If the information conflicts with our beliefs, however, or comes from a person we dislike, we generally label it opinion. In academia, for example, we usually embrace whatever the textbook or the professor declares. We don't always realize that another textbook or another professor may put the same subject in a different perspective.

Fact:

The blood is prepared in the liver and moves through the veins to various organs, where it is consumed.

This "fact" went largely uncontested for fourteen centuries, until 1628, when William Harvey showed how the circulatory system really works.

Opinion:

Washing one's hands before examining women in labor can prevent the spread of puerperal fever.

This "opinion" from Ignaz Semmelweis, vehemently rejected by obstetricians and midwives at the time (1847), is now a life-saving fact.

Why is it so hard to challenge conventional wisdom? Because skeptical questions and maverick views—including those set forth in good faith—place us at risk: the risk of losing a position we have struggled to attain or simply the risk of losing face. History, both medical and general, resounds with stories of individuals who have tried to introduce new ideas but couldn't penetrate the party line. This barrier continues to promote acquiescence and stifle innovation. Consequently, many careers reflect ascent by assent.

For even the most careful speaker or thinker, the ground between fact and opinion often shifts. When fault lines develop, remember: Facts are definitive, permanent, and independent of subjective interpretation; they generate no emotion. Therefore, when we feel strongly about something, we're probably pushing an opinion, not defending a fact.

Today's absolutes are tomorrow's fallacies—and that's a "fact"!

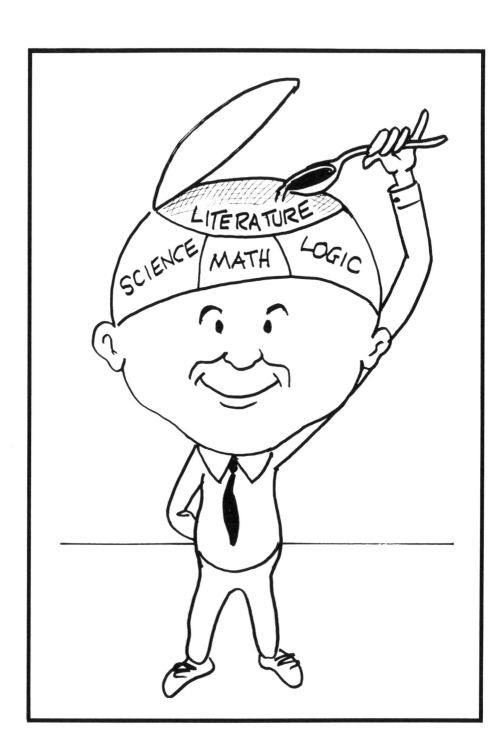

ON BECOMING A FATHEAD*

It's unfortunate that rusty brains do not squeak.
—quoted by McKenzie[1]

As you read this sentence, you are feeding—not your stomach, but your brain.

We always find time to eat. Yet how often do we find time to feast on books and other material outside our line of work? Recently, I feasted on Dashiell Hammett's *The Thin Man.* In it, I joyfully discovered that the thin-bodied hero is awfully fat of mind.

America today is obsessed with the dangers of a fat body. But what good is a well-oiled body if the mind is left to rust? In that light, consider these combinations: thin body/thin mind, thin body/fat mind, fat body/thin mind, and fat body/fat mind. Is the one fitting you the one you deem most fitting?

Achieving and maintaining a thin body or a fat mind necessitate desire, discipline, and dedication. For most of us, a thin body means decreasing our food intake and increasing our physical activity. For *all* of us, however, a fat mind means a diet rich in intellectual calories, devoured regularly and assimilated through repeated mental gymnastics.

When you first saw the title of this essay, you probably flashed back to your schoolyard days. And you probably thought that being called a fathead could never be complimentary. Well, never mind what you had in mind. The fact is, you have *fed* to this point—something only a fathead would do.

*Reprinted by permission from the *Southern Medical Journal* 1989; 82:1265.

REFERENCES

[1]McKenzie EC (Ed.). *14,000 Quips & Quotes for Writers and Speakers.* New York, Greenwich House, 1984, p. 53.

WE DON'T ALWAYS GET
WHAT WE DESERVE*

Getting what we deserve and deserving what we get can be one and the same or two entirely different things. It often boils down to a matter of opinion, and sometimes luck. For example, you work hard (or so you think) and fully expect a raise in pay, but you don't get it. In your eyes, you didn't get what you deserved. But in the eyes of your boss—who had contemplated reducing your pay or actually firing you—you got more than you deserved. Regardless, you're the one who suffers.

Suppose that while driving through a school zone, you ignore a stop sign and exceed the posted speed limit. You definitely deserve a ticket, but you don't get one because no police officer is around. In that instance, you clearly get less than you deserve. And based on the safety threat you pose, the public now suffers.

Consider next the rapists and murderers who never go to jail because of legal technicalities, or who return to the streets early because of overcrowded prisons. Those criminals don't get the punishment they deserve, and they don't deserve the freedom they get. Either way, the public suffers.

*Reprinted by permission from the *Macon Telegraph,* 21 July 1991, 5B.

Though legal roadblocks and penal inadequacies make headlines every day, certain shortcomings in the medical profession fester inconspicuously. Two in particular—sycophancy and silence—deserve more "hollerance" and less tolerance. Sycophancy, better known as buttering up or apple-polishing, characteristically occurs during medical school and postgraduate training. Here, teacher and trainee say and do what each believes the other wants, not necessarily what the other deserves. Both leave these sessions with ego and ignorance intact. As a result, the public suffers.

Sycophancy in private practice can be difficult to spot because its manifestations conform to the "accepted standard of medical care in the community." Primary physicians and consultants tacitly agree not to disagree in order to preserve established referral patterns and guard against malpractice suits. From this courtship, the public suffers.

Silence is the response of many trainees, teachers, and practitioners who know or strongly suspect that one of their colleagues is emotionally disturbed, a substance abuser, a cheater, a liar, or just plain incompetent. The failure to speak out, or reach out, denies the afflicted individuals the corrective measures they deserve and compromises the integrity of those who see but do not say. Sadly, the public suffers.

Buck-passing also plagues the medical profession. Hard-pressed for time and fearful of being sued for overlooking something, many physicians feel compelled to order a myriad of tests and prescribe a multitude of drugs, hoping to detect and alleviate every conceivable ailment. If the patient's condition fails to improve or if results of tests are abnormal, the attending physician may defer to an army of consultants who march in and take over, each managing a different part of the patient's body; nobody manages the whole body. Again, the public suffers.

What about a physician's side of the story? When I hire a person or a company to do a job—repair my fence, install my refrigerator, move my household furnishings, service my car—

inferior work and recurrent delays are common, *if* the "care-provider" shows up at all. The persons responsible for these fiascoes offer the usual excuses but rarely give satisfactory explanations. To make matters worse, they fully expect me to forgive, even condone, their mistakes, oblivious to the fact that in their "care," I suffer.

Yet when these same people seek medical help, they expect perfection. They expect a perfect diagnosis. They expect a perfect cure. With anything less, they are more inclined to sue than to forgive. They view physician error as malpractice and view their own malpractices as mere human frailties. Because of this attitude, physicians suffer.

For this panoply of ills, all of us deserve remedies. But then, we don't always get what we deserve.

DOCTORS AREN'T ORDINARY MORTALS*

> *A physician died after a long and successful career, but when he arrived at the pearly gates of Heaven there was a line and St. Peter refused to be hurried. Accustomed to VIP treatment, the physician went up to St. Peter and asked to be excused from waiting. He was refused on the grounds that Heaven makes no distinction between doctors and ordinary mortals. But while he was waiting, the physician became annoyed when a man in a white coat, stethoscope hanging from his neck and beeper on his belt, came past the line of people and walked straight into Heaven. "Why was he not made to wait also?" exploded the doctor. St. Peter replied: "Actually, that was God himself. He enjoys playing doctor."*
>
> —*The American Rabbi*, Vol. 20, June 1988

True, we doctors *are* accustomed to VIP treatment. Many of us expect it, and some of us seek it. But whether any of us deserves it is another matter.

Regardless of how we stack up in Heaven (assuming we get there), doctors *are* different from "ordinary mortals"—in two "extra-ordinary" ways. We have a license to look at, touch, or probe any part of another person's body. And we can literally bury our mistakes, typically with no outsider ever realizing that we have made them.

These differences make medicine a privileged, yet insulated, profession. If we cherish the privilege and reject the insulation, we doctors won't play God, and God won't have reason to play doctor!

*Reprinted by permission from the *Southern Medical Journal* 1991; 84:550.

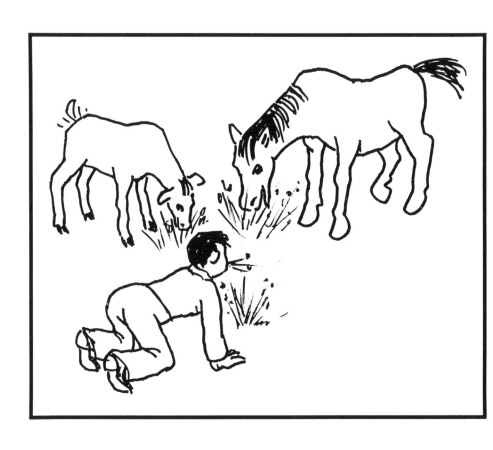

Mairsey Doats and Doesey Doats: Should We?*

If you're not cholesterol-conscious these days, you could be unconscious. Or possibly you never read newspapers or magazines, listen to radio, watch television, shop for groceries, or visit your doctor. Otherwise, you would know that a high serum cholesterol concentration increases the risk of coronary artery disease.[1, 2] You would also know that eating less cholesterol and saturated fats is the safest and cheapest way to decrease your serum cholesterol. But how much do you know about oat bran—the "miracle" food touted to be particularly effective in lowering cholesterol levels?

Oat bran is the ground inner husk of the grain. Oatmeal is the ground product of the whole grain. In contrast to wheat bran, oat bran is largely water soluble. And in general, water-soluble fiber has a greater lipid-lowering effect than does insoluble fiber.[3]

Scientific research leaves no doubt that oat and bean products *can* lower serum cholesterol.[3-13] Buried in all the hoopla, though, are the factors that put this finding in perspective—factors that deserve wider recognition and

*Reprinted by permission from *Houston Medicine* 1989; 5:116–18.

emphasis. The quantity of oat bran and dried beans used in these investigations far exceeds the amount that most people would be likely to eat every day. In one study, for example, 20 hypercholesterolemic men added *100 grams* of oat bran (five muffins and one bowl of hot cereal) or *115 grams* of dried beans ($\frac{1}{2}$ to $\frac{2}{3}$ cups of dried beans or about one pound of cooked beans) daily to their typical high-fat Western diet. After three weeks, the total cholesterol decreased an average of almost 20% with either bran or beans. The LDL-cholesterol decreased about 24%, but the HDL-cholesterol also decreased slightly.[8] Another study of similar design gave nearly identical findings.[11] These experiments show that for hypercholesterolemic people who eat a high-fat diet, the additional consumption of huge amounts of oat bran or dried beans daily can reduce their cholesterol levels considerably.

Another point concerns the usefulness of oat bran for people already adhering to a low-fat diet. After 208 normal volunteers ate such a diet for six weeks, their serum cholesterol concentrations dropped an average of 10.8 mg/dl. Then, 138 of these volunteers added 35 to 40 grams per day of oat bran or oatmeal for six more weeks. Their total cholesterol concentrations decreased an additional 5.4 mg/dl (with oat bran) or 6.5 mg/dl (with oatmeal). The 70 controls continued the low-fat diet for six weeks without oat bran, and their cholesterol levels further decreased 1.2 mg/dl.[6] A similar study gave comparable findings.[13] These observations suggest that for people already eating a low-fat diet, the additional consumption of oat bran in substantial amounts has little effect on serum cholesterol.

The mechanism by which the soluble fiber in oat bran and beans lowers serum cholesterol remains speculative. According to some investigators, soluble fiber may bind cholesterol and bile acids in the intestine and prevent their absorption.[9, 10, 14] Others propose that soluble fiber, through fermentation in the colon, forms short-chain fatty acids, which are absorbed into the portal vein and inhibit synthesis of cholesterol in the liver.[15]

Food manufacturers now put oat bran in breakfast cereals, muffins, bread, bagels, pretzels, animal crackers, graham crackers, fruit bars, wafers, and cookies. But beware! Except for some of the ready-to-eat cereals, most of these products contain less than 5 grams of oat bran per ounce. To get the equivalent of a one-ounce serving of 100% oat bran (20 to 28 grams, depending on the brand[16]), you'd have to finish off a pound of oat-bran animal cookies—but you'd get about 1,100 extra calories in the process. Beware, too, that labels on all sorts of oat bran items, as with those on many prepared foods,[17] can confuse or beguile you. They frequently camouflage how much bran a serving provides, don't always designate clearly what a "serving" is, and never warn that the oils, sugar, and salt in the product could nullify whatever benefit the smidgen of oat bran delivers. And don't delude yourself: "You can't eat your cheesecake with an oat-bran chaser and expect it to clean out your arteries."[18]

Three practical matters merit attention. First, oat bran, like rice, quadruples in volume on cooking. Only small amounts of boiled bran, therefore, may lead to early satiety. Yet, early satiety can be an advantage by reducing the desire or capacity to eat anything else. Second, straight oat bran does not require cooking for consumption, despite what the directions say. It can be eaten as a dry cereal, either plain or flavored with fruits and nuts. This enables you to eat a larger and more effective amount before getting full. Third, quantities of oat bran sufficient to lower the serum cholesterol may cause gaseous distention, flatulence, bulky stools, and increased bowel movements.

In the title of this essay, I posed a question. My answer is, "Yes, if we like oats, and especially if our serum cholesterol is high." But much more important is avoiding the atherogenic demons in our diet—whole milk, cream, butter, cheese, egg yolks, organ meats, animal fats of every kind, and saturated vegetable fats such as palm and coconut oil.[19] Doing that gets to the real "heart" of the matter.

REFERENCES

[1]Gotto AM Jr, Bierman EL, Connor WE, *et al.*, Grundy SM (Ed.). AHA Special Report: Recommendations for treatment of hyperlipidemia in adults. A joint statement of the Nutrition Committee and the Council on Arteriosclerosis. *Circulation* 1984; 69:1065A–90A.

[2]Roberts WC. Atherosclerotic risk factors—Are there ten or is there only one? *Am J Cardiol* 1989; 64:552–54.

[3]Ullrich IH. Evaluation of a high-fiber diet in hyperlipidemia: A review. *J Am Coll Nutrition* 1987; 6:19–25.

[4]Chen W-JL, Anderson JW. Effects of plant fiber in decreasing plasma total cholesterol and increasing high-density lipoprotein cholesterol. *Proc Soc Exp Biol Med* 1979; 162:310–13.

[5]Jenkins DJA, Leeds AR, Newton C, Cummings JH. Effect of pectin, guar gum, and wheat fibre on serum-cholesterol. *Lancet* 1975; 1:1116–17.

[6]Van Horn LV, Liu K, Parker D, *et al.* Serum lipid response to oat product intake with a fat-modified diet. *J Am Diet Assoc* 1986; 86:759–64.

[7]Anderson JW, Gustafson NJ. Hypocholesterolemic effects of oat and bean products. *Am J Clin Nutr* 1988; 48:749–53.

[8]Anderson JW, Story L, Sieling B, *et al.* Hypocholesterolemic effects of oat-bran or bean intake for hypercholesterolemic men. *Am J Clin Nutr* 1984; 40:1146–55.

[9]Kirby RW, Anderson JW, Sieling B, *et al.* Oat-bran intake selectively lowers serum low-density lipoprotein cholesterol concentrations of hypercholesterolemic men. *Am J Clin Nutr* 1981; 34:824–29.

[10]Anderson JW, Tietyen-Clark J. Dietary fiber: Hyperlipidemia, hypertension, and coronary heart disease. *Am J Gastroenterol* 1986; 81:907–19.

[11]Anderson JW, Story L, Sieling B, *et al.* Hypocholesterolemic effects of high-fibre diets rich in water-soluble plant fibres. *J Can Diet Assoc* 1984; 45:140–48.

[12]Mathur KS, Khan MA, Sharma RD. Hypocholesterolaemic effect of Bengal gram: A long-term study in man. *Br Med J* 1968; 1:30–31.

[13]Van Horn L, Emidy LA, Liu K, *et al.* Short report: Serum lipid response to a fat-modified, oatmeal-enhanced diet. *Prev Med* 1988; 17:377–86.

[14]Kay RM. Dietary fiber. *J Lipid Res* 1982; 23:221–42.

[15]Chen W-JL, Anderson JW, Jennings D. Propionate may mediate the hypocholesterolemic effects of certain soluble plant fibers in cholesterol-fed rats. *Proc Soc Exp Biol Med* 1984; 175:215–18.

[16]Oat bran for lowering blood lipids. *The Medical Letter, Inc.* 1988; 30 (December 2):111–12.

[17]Kessler DA. The federal regulation of food labeling: Promoting foods to prevent disease. *N Engl J Med* 1989; 321:717–25.

[18]Van Horn LV, quoted in *The Houston Post,* Houston, Texas, September 10, 1989, pp. F1, F9.

[19]Blum CB, Levy RI. Current therapy for hypercholesterolemia. *JAMA* 1989; 261:3582–87.

HOSPITAL CARE: HELPFUL OR HARMFUL?

During a recent stay in a Houston hospital, the wife of a local ophthalmologist received an injection of penicillin—a common, sometimes life-saving event. In her case, however, the injection became life-threatening. She sweated profusely, her heart raced, and her eyes swelled. In addition, she had trouble breathing, and her blood pressure dropped. Fortunately, with appropriate subsequent treatment, she recovered completely. Nonetheless, both the ophthalmologist and his wife remain astonished that such a mistake occurred—the wife had explicitly told the attending nurse of her allergy to penicillin. How could the nurse have forgotten?

According to the Harvard Medical Practice Study, published several months ago in *The New England Journal of Medicine,* adverse events are frequent enough during hospitalization to warrant the serious attention of everybody, not just members of the medical community. The authors of that study defined an adverse event as an injury that resulted from in-hospital care and that prolonged the patient's stay, produced a disability at the time of discharge, or both. They also determined which of these events resulted from negligence—defined by them as "care that fell below the standard expected of physicians in their community."

*Reprinted by permission from *The Houston Post,* 16 April 1991, A-11.

The study involved a review of 30,121 randomly selected records from 51 randomly selected acute care, nonpsychiatric hospitals in New York state. It provides for the first time statistically reliable estimates of adverse events, including the events due to negligence. The numbers are sobering:

• A total of 98,609 adverse events occurred among 2,671,863 patients.

• Negligence accounted for 27,179 of the adverse events.

• Of the adverse events caused by negligence, 877 led to permanent total disability, and 6,895 resulted in death.

• From the adverse events not related to negligence, permanent total disability developed in 2,550 patients, and 13,451 patients died.

These findings prompt a frightening conclusion: in-hospital medical management injures a substantial number of patients, and nearly one-third of the injuries arise from substandard care.

Though the kinds of adverse events in that study varied considerably, drug-related complications predominated. To learn more about such drug-related events, a group of investigators in Los Angeles recently analyzed 122 hospital records, comparing the medication histories written in those records with medication histories obtained from the patients by a research staff. They defined an error as either the failure to record a medication the patient claimed to use or the recording of a medication the patient denied using. Almost two-thirds of the records contained at least one error, and one-fifth of them had three errors or more. Errors of omission were evident in more than half the records and errors of commission in nearly one-fourth the records. Obviously, inaccurate medication histories make medication errors more likely, if not inevitable.

Can we rectify these medication errors, these adverse events, these all-too-frequent mishaps of hospital care? I believe we can, but only with concerted, cooperative efforts by everyone on the health-care team—physicians, nurses, administrators, pharmacists, laboratory technicians, medical records librarians, dietitians, social workers, maintenance personnel, and security agents. All of these people, in one way or another, influence the welfare of hospitalized patients.

If we are to minimize adverse events in the hospital, we must demonstrate compassion, commitment, candor, and common sense. We must also develop and implement in-hospital educational systems, including those designed for patients. We must insist on strict credentialing of all physicians applying for staff privileges; pay more than lip service to the peer-review process; and strive for *quality* in our quality-assurance programs. And if all this seems too much, try becoming a patient in a hospital. That's the surest way to appreciate what patients really go through.

We in the medical community have an ethical obligation to do all we can to prevent medical mishaps and to make hospital care helpful, not harmful. In the wake of the Harvard Medical Practice Study, let us acknowledge that errors in medical care are costly—in time, in money, in livelihood, in lives. They further inflate the ever-spiraling cost of health care; we simply can't afford them any longer.

MY WIFE'S BACK*

If you're wondering about that title, my wife didn't leave me. She has a problem with her back—recurrent subluxation of the sacroiliac joint.

The difficulty started abruptly six years ago while my wife was dressing. On raising her right leg to step into her skirt, she experienced excruciating pain across her lower back and collapsed onto the floor. She spent the next three weeks in bed on a heating pad, loaded with analgesics, sedatives, and muscle relaxants. Besides pain, she complained of inability to stand straight and of tilting to the right. Thereafter, she suffered many similar episodes, all of which incapacitated her from four to seven or more days. During each attack, she tilted to the right, and her pain invariably was most intense over the right sacroiliac joint. The pain never radiated. Wearing a back brace or attempting conventional back exercises aggravated the pain. Repeated physical examinations showed no neurological deficits. A gamut of laboratory studies, including bone scans and films of the lumbosacral spine and pelvis, showed no abnormality. Computed tomography and magnetic resonance imaging (MRI) of the lumbosacral spine demonstrated a bulging disc at L4-5 on the right. Her diagnoses alternated between low back strain and disc disease.

*Reprinted by permission from *Houston Medicine* 1990; 6:43–44.

With time, the episodes became more frequent, and she and I became more frustrated and desperate. Seemingly innocuous movements—sneezing, getting in and out of cars, bending over to pick up a newspaper, twisting to load the dishwasher, reaching for a book—sometimes caused her back to "go out." Physical intimacy with each other always increased her discomfort and commonly provoked an attack. Even between attacks, her back ached, forcing her to move slowly and cautiously.

Eventually, the pain and tilt became relentless, but a follow-up MRI showed *regression* of the previously documented bulging disc. Baffled, I sought Dr. James E. Butler's opinion. He diagnosed recurrent subluxation of the right sacroiliac joint and referred my wife to the physical therapist who had taught him how to recognize the disorder. The therapist, in turn, taught her how to reduce the subluxation by herself.

My wife's back still "goes out." But now instead of requiring days in bed to recover, she needs just a few minutes to put the joint back into place. The maneuver usually gives prompt and complete relief. On four occasions, however, when the maneuver didn't work, the joint later went back into place by itself, suddenly. Three times this happened during sleep. My wife rolled to one side, awakened with severe pain, felt and heard a "pop," then was pain free. The same sequence—pain, "pop," no pain—occurred once while she was making a bed.

Though her sacroiliac joint remains unstable and cure is nowhere in sight, my wife's back—back from having relentless pain; back from being frustrated and filled with despair; back from expecting and fearing spinal surgery; and back, almost, to her normal self.

Surgical Standby Arrangements for Elective Percutaneous Transluminal Coronary Angioplasty*

Should the backup surgeon necessarily be within the institution during elective percutaneous transluminal coronary angioplasty (PTCA)? Should a cardiac operating room be kept open during the procedure? To what extent do insurance companies pay hospital costs and physicians' fees for standby time? Is the standby arrangement a high legal risk?

These questions and others related to surgical standby arrangements for elective PTCA stimulated a lively discussion at a recent meeting of the Medical Staff Executive Committee of my hospital (HCA Medical Center Hospital in Houston).† The committee selected me to investigate this matter because I am the hospital's educational coordinator and am neither a cardiologist nor a surgeon. Accordingly, I contacted national organizations for their guidelines or recommendations; looked

---

*Reprinted by permission from the *Southern Medical Journal* 1990; 83:1459–62.

†Some of the material in this article tends toward the technical. Its genesis was, after all, in the context of a medical staff committee meeting. Nonetheless, the article gives lay readers background information on PTCAs that would otherwise be unavailable—information that could be crucial in the medical future of some readers.—ED.

into current PTCA policies at Houston-area hospitals outside the Texas Medical Center; reviewed the pertinent medical literature; gathered relevant legal and insurance data; and talked with prominent cardiologists, cardiac surgeons, and anesthesiologists across the country.

National Guidelines and Position Papers

The organizations contacted were: the Joint Commission on Accreditation of Healthcare Organizations (JCAHO), American Hospital Association, American Board of Anesthesiology, American Board of Thoracic Surgery, Society of Thoracic Surgeons, American College of Physicians (ACP), and American College of Cardiology/American Heart Association (ACC/AHA). Of these, only the last two address this problem officially.

The ACP position paper,[1] published in 1983, simply says: "An experienced and highly skilled thoracic cardiovascular surgical team must be available as backup whenever this technique [PTCA] is done." By contrast, the ACC/AHA guidelines for PTCA[2(pp. 490–91)] are more detailed and specific:

> An experienced cardiovascular surgical team should be available within the institution for emergency surgery for all angioplasty procedures. . . . there should be no exception to this requirement. . . . [Nevertheless, the guidelines footnote an exception:] "Within the institution" is generally intended to mean within the same hospital. In those instances in which two adjacent hospitals are physically connected such that emergency transport by stretcher or gurney can be achieved rapidly and effectively, the transport of patients between the two hospitals for emergency cardiac surgical services would not be viewed as "off site."

William L. Winters, Jr., M.D., a member of the ACC/AHA guidelines subcommittee and president of the American College of Cardiology, told me that observance of the ACC/AHA guidelines has relaxed substantially throughout America. He emphasized that the PTCA policy for a particular hospital will depend primarily on factors specific to that hospital.

Houston-Area Policies on Surgical Standby

Of six representative Houston-area hospitals located outside the Texas Medical Center, five require the backup surgeon and pump team to be in the hospital during the procedure. One, however, permits the surgeon to wait in an adjacent professional building.

Scope of the Problem

In a 1988 report, Parsonnet *et al.*[3] reviewed fifteen articles (including their own) comprising 15,802 PTCA failures. They found that 902 patients (5.7%) required emergency operation. Follow-up on 868 of these patients showed that 51 (5.9%) died after the operation. But the true incidence of emergency operations after failed PTCA is lower than the 5.7% they reported, because not all of the articles they reviewed distinguished between "emergent" and "urgent" operations. "Emergent" operations are those done immediately after PTCA because of hemodynamic instability, intractable chest pain, ominous ECG changes, or coronary artery occlusion, dissection, or perforation. "Urgent" operations are those done within twenty-four hours of PTCA because of therapeutic failure or stable complications.

Predictors of In-hospital Mortality after Elective PTCA

The following factors continue to show a multivariate association with in-hospital mortality after elective PTCA.[2(p. 495), 3, 4]

Clinical:

1. Extent of coronary artery disease: single vessel, 0.2%; double vessel, 0.9%; triple vessel, 2.2%; left main coronary artery, 8.1%
2. Severe proximal lesion of the left anterior descending coronary artery
3. Unstable or new onset angina
4. Cardiogenic shock
5. History of congestive heart failure
6. Previous myocardial infarction or bypass surgery

7. Age 65 years or older
8. Female gender
9. History of hypertension
10. Diabetes mellitus

Procedural:

11. Myocardial infarction, ventricular fibrillation

Time between Call for Surgical Intervention and Revascularization

Minimizing the duration of myocardial ischemia after failed PTCA is obviously important, especially in terms of patient survival.[5] Yet reports on failed PTCA do not routinely correlate this time factor with mortality. In fact, the actual ischemic time is not clear in many of the studies.[6] Rarely mentioned, for example, is the estimated time spent in the catheterization laboratory attempting to manage the complication before deciding to call for surgical help.

In a report by Murphy *et al.,*[7] the time from onset of severe chest pain in the catheterization laboratory to completed coronary artery grafting ranged from 75 to 210 minutes. Brahos and associates[8] indicated that "operative intervention was initiated within 15 minutes in some patients in unstable condition, but within two hours in most circumstances." Jones *et al.*[9] said: "Two hours is about as fast as one can get a patient from the catheterization laboratory and have him or her completely revascularized." And according to James T. Willerson, M.D., a leading cardiologist, "Usually about 40 minutes to an hour elapses between the decision to operate and the surgeon's 'first cut' " (oral communication, July 1990).

Customary delays of this magnitude prompted Bonchek[10] to take issue with the ACC/AHA requirement that a backup surgeon be present within the institution: "In my own experience, a slightly longer interval to revascularization has seemed much less important in determining the extent of myocardial injury after failed PTCA than has the presence or absence of residual patency in the offending coronary artery, because it is the residual coronary lumen that regulates perfusion of the jeopardized myocardium." He also pointed out that the German Society of Cardiology has a policy statement about surgical backup that permits PTCA to be done in one hospital with support from a standby team in another hospital geographically separate but close by.

A subsequent report from Belfast, Ireland,[11] supported Bonchek's argument. In a hospital that had no on-site cardiac surgical coverage, twelve patients who had PTCA required urgent surgical revascularization. They were transported safely 2.4 km to another hospital that did have cardiac surgical coverage; none of these patients died. The mean delay before revascularization was 268 minutes (range, 180 to 390 minutes). For patients who had PTCA in the hospital that did have cardiac surgical coverage, the delay in revascularization was virtually identical at 273 minutes (range, 108 to 420 minutes). The principal cause of the delay in both patient populations was "the wait for a cardiac operating theatre to become available and not the transfer time between hospitals. . . . The absence of immediate surgical help did not influence the outcome in any patient."

Availability of Cardiac Operating Room

A recent survey of 89 hospitals wherein coronary angioplasty and coronary artery grafting are done regularly showed that 64% maintain an open operating room during PTCA.[12] Twenty-four percent use the "next available room" method. Eight percent either did not describe their usual arrangement or indicated that it varied. Four percent had no formal standby arrangement. And 29% modified their usual standby arrangements when they had unusual or high-risk PTCA cases. As experience with PTCA accumulates, more and more hospitals are adopting the "next available room" approach.[6-8, 12]

Legal Data

A Lexis (computerized) search of the legal literature conducted in the Hospital Corporation of America corporate offices showed that, as of July 1990, no lawsuits related to surgical standby arrangements during PTCA have arisen in the United States. This fact is important to hospital administrators and cardiac surgeons[9] concerned about the legal aspects of this matter.

Insurance Data

Third-party payors are reluctant to pay for surgical standby services.[6, 12] As a result, these costs are sometimes absorbed as a large surcharge on other cardiac surgical procedures, on catheterization laboratory fees, or on the care of all hospital patients.[5, 12] In a detailed study of 699 PTCAs for which simultaneous surgical standby was available, Wilson et al.[5] found that the surgeons stood by for more than 2,500 hours (an average of 3.6 hours per PTCA), and the actual cost of surgical standby for each attempted PTCA exceeded $1,700. Considering that 227,000 patients had PTCA in this country in 1988[13] and that fewer than 5% of such cases require emergency bypass grafting, surgical standby arrangements are not cost effective, and they waste lots of professional time and talent.

I obtained information from five insurance carriers regarding payment for surgical standby services. Blue Cross/ Blue Shield responded: "In most conditions, if no care is rendered to the patient, there is no reimbursement." John Hancock Company indicated that it does reimburse for surgical standby. Equicor, Hartford, and Aetna insurance companies were unable to give definitive answers. With regard to Medicare Part B reimbursement, the following ruling appeared in the September 1986 Medicare Bulletin:

> In terms of the surgical stand-by team which is available when PTCA is performed, it does not appear that the physician members of this team perform identifiable patient care services unless the patient undergoes bypass surgery.

For example, the immediate availability of the cardiac surgeon in the operating room does not constitute a reimbursable physician's service. Therefore, no Part B payments may be recognized to any physician member of the stand-by team.[6]

Comment

Though surgical standby arrangements vary considerably across the country, two things about them are clear: none is cost effective, and none to date has led to a lawsuit. But whether the backup surgeon should be within the institution during PTCA and whether a cardiac operating room should be kept open are issues that remain unsettled. Nevertheless, in my discussions with cardiologists, anesthesiologists, and cardiac surgeons across the country, the consensus was that cardiac surgeons who wish to remain outside the institution during PTCA should be allowed to do so—provided they get no farther away than "next door, across the street, or 10 minutes by foot."

Now that cardiologists have PTCA at their disposal, more and more of them are encroaching on territory that once belonged solely to cardiac surgeons. Not surprisingly, therefore, a certain amount of ill will has developed.[5, 9, 12] In a survey of eighty-nine hospitals that regularly conduct PTCA and coronary artery grafting, Cameron et al.[12] found that 37% of the surgeons (33/89) were dissatisfied with their standby arrangements. The most common complaints concerned possibly inappropriate selection of patients for PTCA, poor communication with cardiologists regarding high-risk patients, waste of operating room resources, and inadequate compensation. During my investigation, some cardiac surgeons complained that the cardiologists give them no input in determining a mutually convenient time for the angioplasty. Others told me they commonly stand by because they are expected to, and that in such circumstances, their "consultation" note is noncommittal: "I have been asked to serve as surgical standby should the need for emergency operation arise during this PTCA. I agree to do so." Some also said that even when they disagree with PTCA in a particular case, they still stand by, fearful of losing patient referrals if they don't.

To improve current standby practices, some hospitals schedule PTCAs around noon or later, when operating room activities are generally winding down.[9, 12] This approach helps ensure the shortest waiting period between a PTCA mishap and an available operating room. It also maximizes surgical resources and minimizes tensions.

Ullyot[6] offers a selective approach wherein patients at particularly high risk could be seen in consultation by the surgeon before PTCA. If the surgeon agreed to angioplasty, formal standby with an operating room held open could be provided. Under this arrangement, most patients would be managed without formal standby, and surgical consultation would be sought when a complication occurs—as with any other medical procedure carrying risk. "Omnipresent surgical standby poised to respond instantly and automatically to iatrogenic injury, however, is no longer appropriate for a technology well beyond its developmental stages."[6]

I think we should concentrate more on *preventing* the complications of PTCA. *Who* does the angioplasty and *why* are certainly as important as who stands by and where. Consequently, we should insist on strict credentialing of all cardiologists seeking coronary angioplasty privileges.[2(pp. 499–500), 14, 15] Once they obtain such privileges, we should require these cardiologists to meet established guidelines for maintaining competence in PTCA.[15] We should also require the anesthesiologist and backup surgeon to provide preangioplasty evaluations in *all* elective PTCAs, including those thought to carry minimal risk for the patient. Such evaluations should include examining the patient, reviewing the pertinent studies, and discussing the potential bypass grafting with the patient. This approach affords the anesthesiologist and cardiac surgeon the kind of firsthand presurgical information they would need to render the best possible care if an emergency operation were to become necessary. It would improve communication between everyone involved and, in some instances, prevent ill-advised PTCAs. And these evaluations would be reimbursable. Yet today, only about one-third of patients undergoing PTCA receive preangioplasty evaluation by a surgeon, an anesthesiologist, or both.[12] So in most of the cases, we are giving the cardiologist unbridled authority to immobilize a cardiac surgeon, an anesthesiologist, a pump team, and an operating room.

Isn't it time we tightened the "reigns"?

REFERENCES

[1]Health and Public Policy Committee, American College of Physicians. Percutaneous transluminal angioplasty. *Ann Intern Med* 1983; 99:864–69.

[2]American College of Cardiology/American Heart Association Task Force on Assessment of Diagnostic and Therapeutic Cardiovascular Procedures (Subcommittee on Percutaneous Transluminal Coronary Angioplasty). Guidelines for percutaneous transluminal coronary angioplasty. *Circulation* 1988; 78:486–502.

[3]Parsonnet V, Fisch D, Gielchinsky I, *et al.* Emergency operation after failed angioplasty. *J Thorac Cardiovasc Surg* 1988; 96:198–203.

[4]Holmes DR Jr, Holubkov R, Vlietstra RE, *et al.* Comparison of complications during percutaneous transluminal coronary angioplasty from 1977 to 1981 and from 1985 to 1986: The National Heart, Lung, and Blood Institute Percutaneous Transluminal Coronary Angioplasty Registry. *J Am Coll Cardiol* 1988; 12:1149–55.

[5]Wilson JM, Dunn EJ, Wright CB, *et al.* The cost of simultaneous surgical standby for percutaneous transluminal coronary angioplasty. *J Thorac Cardiovasc Surg* 1986; 91:362–70.

[6]Ullyot DJ. Surgical standby for percutaneous coronary angioplasty. *Circulation* 1987; 76 (suppl 3):149–52.

[7]Murphy DA, Craver JM, Jones EL, *et al.* Surgical revascularization following unsuccessful percutaneous transluminal coronary angioplasty. *J Thorac Cardiovasc Surg* 1982; 84:342–48.

[8]Brahos GJ, Baker NH, Ewy HG, *et al.* Aortocoronary bypass following unsuccessful PTCA: experience in 100 consecutive patients. *Ann Thorac Surg* 1985; 40:7–10.

[9]Jones EL, Craver JM, Grüntzig AR, *et al.* Percutaneous transluminal coronary angioplasty: role of the surgeon. *Ann Thorac Surg* 1982; 34:493–503.

[10]Bonchek LI: Should surgical support within the same institution be required for percutaneous transluminal coronary angioplasty? *Ann Thorac Surg* 1989; 48:159–60.

[11]Richardson SG, Morton P, Murtagh JG, *et al.* Management of acute coronary occlusion during percutaneous, transluminal coronary angioplasty: experience of complications in a hospital without on site facilities for cardiac surgery. *Br Med J* 1990; 300:355–58.

[12]Cameron DE, Stinson DC, Greene PS, *et al.* Surgical standby for percutaneous transluminal coronary angioplasty: a survey of patterns of practice. *Ann Thorac Surg* 1990; 50:35–39.

[13]Ullyot DJ. Surgical standby for coronary angioplasty. *Ann Thorac Surg* 1990; 50:3–4.

[14]Cowley MJ, King S III, and the Committee on Interventional Cardiology, The Society for Cardiac Angiography. Guidelines for credentialing and facilities for performance of coronary angioplasty. *Cathet Cardiovasc Diagn* 1988; 15:136–38.

[15]Ryan TJ, Klocke FJ, Reynolds WA. AHA Medical/Scientific Statement: clinical competence in percutaneous transluminal coronary angioplasty. a statement for physicians from the ACP/ACC/AHA task force on clinical privileges in cardiology. *Circulation* 1990; 81:2041–46.

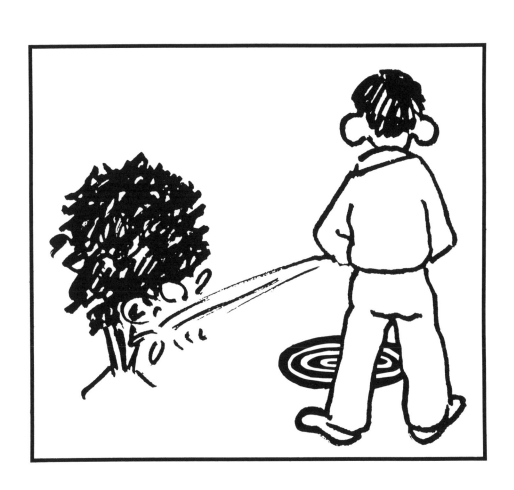

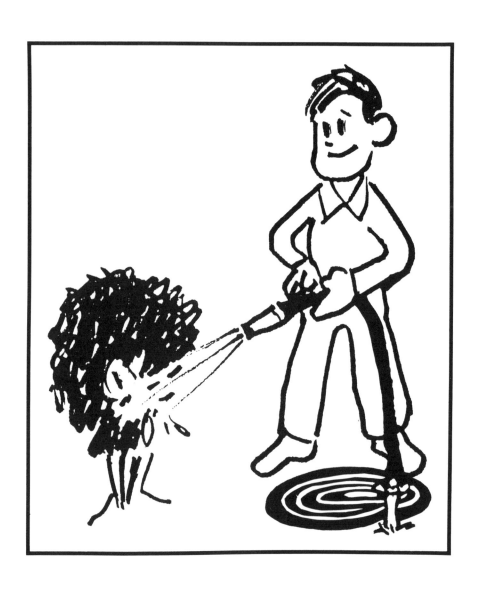

PEEING IS BELIEVING*

As a full-time medical educator, I often use analogies to make my point. In the past, when I seriously doubted a house officer's diagnosis, I would say, "That diagnosis is about as likely as my peeing in the ocean and expecting the tide to rise." Now, when I spout that analogy I secretly smile, because my ability to raise the tide has improved markedly. Here's why.

For almost a year I thought I had recurring prostatitis. I was having intermittent signs of urinary irritation—frequency, urgency, and terminal burning—accompanied at times by many white blood cells in my prostatic fluid. Obstructive manifestations were minimal, in comparison. My prostate gland felt normal to physical examination, but on transrectal ultrasonography, it appeared mildly enlarged in the central zone. When various therapies for prostatitis failed and my symptoms worsened, cystoscopy became necessary. It showed prostatic hypertrophy causing substantial obstruction of the bladder neck and moderate trabeculation of the bladder wall.

To pee or not to pee? That was the question. After weighing my alternatives, I took the "roto-rooter" route. Happily, everything came out all right, and I recaptured my fountain of youth.

I conclude that an older man's best friend is not his dog, but his urologist. Thanks to my urologist, I'm void of discomfort and back in the flow, my troubled waters calmed.

*Reprinted by permission from the *Southern Medical Journal* 1991; 84:488.

THE SICK SENSE SYNDROME*

Have you ever had some sense knocked into you and out of you at the same time? Well, I have. It happened two years ago on my daily run. I argued with a car and lost. As a result, I suffered widespread injuries, including a fractured skull, subdural hematoma, and hemorrhage throughout both temporal and frontal lobes of my brain. What got knocked into me was a heightened sense of awareness—awareness that life is like a beautiful piece of crystal: precious, but fragile. What got knocked out of me were my senses of taste and smell.

The accident convinced me that we tend to take our five senses for granted, at least until one of them gets sick. When that happens, the victim has what I call the "sick sense syndrome." It can affect our sense of sight, hearing, touch, taste, or smell.

*Reprinted by permission from the *Southern Medical Journal* 1989; 82:1155.

But the most common type of sensory failure—the one that harms all of us the most—is failure to use our *common* sense. I call that the "sick sixth sense syndrome."

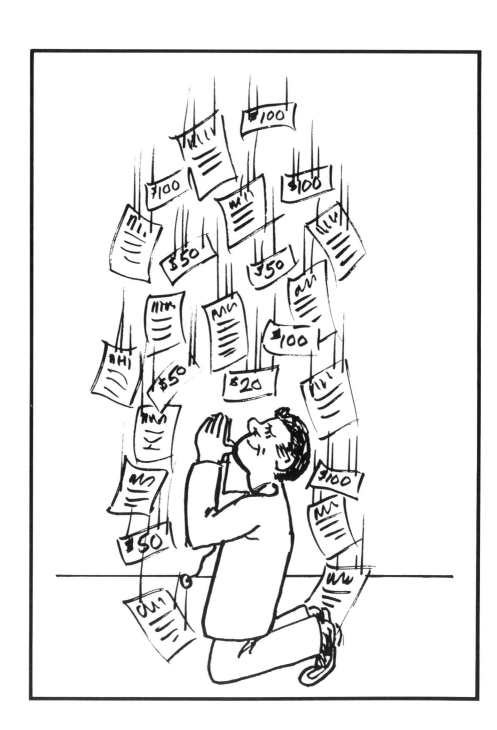

SNACKS TO SECURE SOLVENCY OR CONFESSIONS OF AN EDITOR-IN-CHIEF*

Foreword

Attachment to a single letter of the alphabet may seem, to some, strangely fetishistic behavior. In the right hands, though, single letters may assume a talismanic power. Nathaniel Hawthorne and, more recently, John Updike based entire novels on single letters. And witness the mileage that George Bush recently got out of loudly proclaiming the *l* word and then daring Michael Dukakis to use it in anything above a whisper.

Or take the case of Georges Perec—most recently known for authorship of *Life, a User's Manual*, who in one novel used every vowel but *e* and then in another used only *e*. Perec, having constructed a 1,200-word palindrome, surely had language powers "far beyond those of ordinary men."

A few more such exercises as this and Dr. Fred may well have delivered his first modernist novel. What he has done here, besides depriving us of breath, is to challenge our vocabularies. How he settled on the letter *f* is a matter for his biographers to unearth. My own suspicion is that he began at *a* and interviewed candidates until he found one that suited him. However, I don't rule out that, as a marathoner, Dr. Fred began at *z* and made his way backward—slowly, very slowly.

*Reprinted by permission from the *Southern Medical Journal* 1989; 82:632.

Beneath all the filigree with *f,* Dr. Fred has a nugget of realistic advice for journal supporters of all kinds to feed on.

Susan M. Carini, Managing Editor
Mercer University Press, Macon, Georgia

Fanatical fitness freaks like me frankly fear being fubsy, flabby, or fatigued. So, first and foremost, we furiously frown on foods that fatten our frames, forever fabricating and finagling ways to foil fiddling with them. There is, however, a famous but flagrantly forbidden form of fondant that I'm fond of; and I fight for it frequently, fiercely, feverishly, and ferociously.

Friends, if you find this fancy work far-fetched, frenzied, foozling, funky, fuzzy, fishy, farcical, frivolous, flippant, flighty, feckless, fey, facetious, fatuous, faineant, fulsome, futile, fustian, full of folly, fathomless, a fardel, a foible, a fable, or a forum for flapdoodle, forgive me. Don't forget, forsake, fustigate, fulminate, flog, flay, or fillet me. The foodstuff I fantasticate is M&Ms.

Forsooth, M&Ms are the fulcrum from which folios flourish; they furnish the flavor all editors favor. Without M&Ms, journals become flimsy; readers' fervor fizzles; and fate finally finishes the floundering, fugacious, fundless, futureless fiasco. That's a firm, fundamental, and formidable fact—free of frosting, frills, foofaraw, and flimflammery.

Folks, should you still fail to figure out or follow the fabric of this forensic filibuster, don't fret, fuss, fidget, fume, fleer, faint, feed me flak, or get fractious. Fortunately, I can flat-out forestall the fostering and fomenting of any feud, friction, fracas, or fisticuffs between us, freshen your focus, furbish your faculties, fulgurate your frustrations, and fix your fractured feelings—all with facility, fidelity, and fraternity. For I'm not a fastuous fink who feloniously frolics. Nor am I a finicky fud who foolishly fudges or a full-fledged four-flusher who fiendishly flip-flops. I function, instead, as a fastidious but fallible fellow with a flair for fairness who will forfeit formality, forgo further footle, fess up forthrightly, and fast forge this fandango to fruition.

Finale: In the publishing field, M&Ms are Manuscripts & Money, the fare editors forage for frantically and feast on felicitously when face-to-face with famine.

Finis.

ALCOHOLICS SYNONYMOUS*

The two of us are addicts in every sense of the word. We can't say "no," we crave our "substance" daily, and if we miss a "fix," we suffer withdrawal reactions. Yet, in contrast to most addicts, we're proud of our addictions and practice them openly. We even recommend them. They don't threaten society's welfare; they cost more time than money; and the longer we continue them, the better off we are. Our siren songs follow.

Addict No. 1

I am a 61-year-old physician and full-time medical educator. In 1966, I weighed 200 pounds, ate a high-fat diet, smoked cigarettes and cigars, and had a few cocktails before my evening meal. The only exercise I got was jumping to conclusions or flying off the handle. I was a mainstream American.

About that time, evidence was accumulating that physical inactivity, smoking, and eating too much of the wrong kinds of food were all mileposts on the road to coronary artery disease. Not favoring that trip, I decided to restructure my life-style. I reduced my intake of fats and calories, gave up

*Reprinted by permission from the *Houston Chronicle,* 29 July 1990, 1E.
Susan M. Carini is coauthor of this article.—ED.

tobacco, and eliminated my nightly cocktails. My reward was losing 50 pounds. Encouraged, I started to run regularly and have since covered almost 140,000 miles, averaging 15-20 miles every day.

I don't run high mileage just for my health. I *like* to run. Furthermore, my daily run gives me three to four uninterrupted hours to think—hours during which I can concentrate on work-related issues, on family matters, on manuscripts that I'm writing, or on things I plan to do. It's a time I covet for reflection and introspection.

My world is also larger, thanks to running. Because I run on city streets at midday, I see life from myriad standpoints. I see construction workers, delivery persons, gardeners, children of all ages, pets of all types, and a host of sports enthusiasts. When I visit another city or country, I run where tour buses never go and see things that other visitors never see.

Many runners experience a "high" during their runs. I don't. My "high" begins immediately after each run and lasts until the next day. It is a combination of feelings. I feel grateful to God for His many blessings and to my family for understanding me. I feel privileged to have a job that allows me to run when I want to. And I feel fulfilled, because each run strengthens my body, sharpens my mind, and enriches me spiritually.

Twenty-four years ago, I made a decision. That decision may not have added years to my life, but it has certainly added life to my years.

Addict No. 2

I am the managing editor of a university press. Terminology is already at hand to describe a wretch like me: bibliophile, and the infinitely more sinister, bibliomaniac. But why not devise a more accessible term, the sort that Tom Q. Thumb can stick his lexical finger in? Such a term might be book drunk.

On most days I am either in a bookstore or pinned between the pages of a winsome catalog of books. When I forsake both and am a guest in other people's homes, I read the spines of their books. When I sigh approvingly, it is not about their orange flambé, but rather about their current stock of reading material. In houses with Danielle Steel on the pool deck, I make my excuses early. In dusty, airless houses featuring John Cheever novels, I could stay forever.

During walks with knowing friends, I am steered down streets devoid of any bookstores. Mean streets. (Mean friends.) Eager to prevent my fall, these friends treat bookstores as if they were tattoo parlors—places of ill repute where I could do myself harm. Indeed, even members of my family have not given me a book since 1962, presumably to avoid complicity.

And speaking of families, I sometimes fantasize—between page turns—about forsaking the single life. Once married, I could, for instance, "lift" my husband's golf-club fund and buy him 24 books on the same subject, which is twice the number of cumbersome clubs he would have received. I know instinctively that our child would willingly sacrifice six months' worth of Batman cereal for an original edition of *The Hobbit*.

At work there is no sneaking, none of the usual desperation that leads to stuffing Waldenbooks purchases in a J.C. Penney bag. At the office they ask me to read, ask me to keep my horizons broad and my mind open to the ever-revolving catherine wheel of knowledge and opinion. Imagine.

Coda

The bad news is that addictions are rampant these days. The good news is that not all of them are harmful.

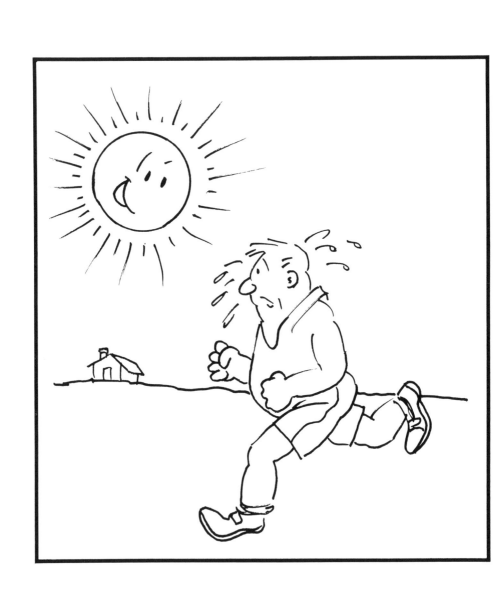

FOR RUNNERS ONLY

Between 70 and 90 miles, mental strain predominated. I hated everyone who had dreamed up four ultramarathon events and a massive relay race on the same course at the same time. I also resented the relay runners. Their task seemed miniscule compared with mine. They seemed to threaten bodily injury whenever they came whizzing by me, so I asked my partner to run directly behind me as a shield. Even my helpers irritated me whenever they tried to make me drink.

My sensory perception was distorted too. Every time my partner's foot struck a particular manhole cover, the clang startled and upset me. But the honking of cars, the noise of the crowd cheering the relay runners, the heat, the humidity, and my nagging nausea all seemed dulled by my obsessive concentration on finishing. At this point runners and spectators began to shout, "Hang in there, you're looking good." I thanked them for their encouragement, but I knew what I really looked like.

H.L.F.
—in "One Hundred Miles, The First Time"

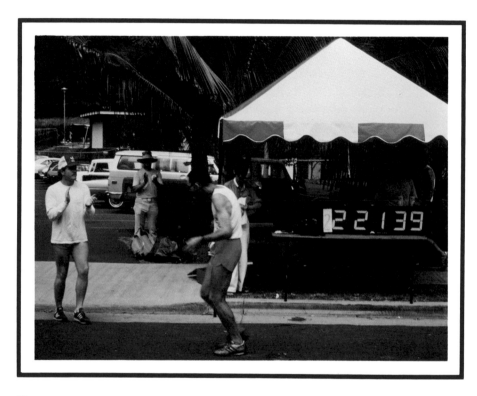

The author finishing his first 100-mile run (time: 22 hours, 21 minutes, 39 seconds), Honolulu, Hawaii, 26–27 May 1979.

ONE HUNDRED MILES, THE FIRST TIME*

Why would a man just shy of his fiftieth birthday try to run 100 miles? For me, the answer begins in 1966, when I started a long-distance running program. Three years later I ran my first marathon. During the next eight years I averaged 100 miles a week and ran 25 marathons, hoping always to break three hours. The closest I got was 3:08:23. By December 1977, I had logged 55,000 miles. At that time an injury forced me to run a marathon slower than usual. I enjoyed the race and felt fresh at the end, so I decided to try an ultramarathon.

In February 1978, I entered the Gulf AAU 50-Mile Championship. Of twenty-six starters, I placed eleventh in 6:51:47. Three months later, in Honolulu, I was the second of seven finishers in the Primo 100 Kilometer run, with a time of 10:42:34. These two experiences convinced me that although I couldn't run fast, I could run far. Now I wanted a 100-miler and aimed for the Primo 100 Mile Race scheduled for May 1979 in Honolulu.

For the next eleven months I averaged twenty miles a day in single, midday workouts, at a pace between 8 and 10 minutes a mile. I craved and ate large amounts of meat, especially beef, with fruit, nuts, and bran for dessert. I also took one multivitamin tablet, three to four grams of vitamin C,

*Reprinted by permission from *Ultrarunning* 1982; January-February:14–15.

and 4,000 IU of vitamin E daily, because that dose and combination of vitamins seemed to keep me free of muscle stiffness and soreness.

In February 1979, I finished third among eleven at the Gulf AAU 100 km championship, in a time of 9:50:19. Soon afterwards I began to lengthen some of my training runs, and for a month I averaged 160 miles a week, running many thirty-milers and one forty-miler. Two weeks before the race, I cut back drastically and totaled only thirty-seven miles in the final six days. Forty-eight hours before the race, I stopped eating roughage and loaded up on animal protein and fat because these foods seemed to boost my endurance.

My goal was to finish the 100 miles, though I wanted to break twenty-four hours and even hoped to break twenty.

The race involved running twenty-five times around a flat, four-mile loop that took in sidewalks, residential streets, and a major highway. In addition to my event, which began at 4 P.M., a 100-km race would start at 8 P.M., a fifty-mile run at 11 P.M., and a fifty-km run at 2 A.M., all on the same course. Then, at 6 A.M., 6,000 relay runners would take off, each running one four-mile loop.

I had five helpers: my wife Judy; two of my running partners, Mark Scheid and Walter Isle; and their wives, Mary and Brenda. The plan was for me to run the first twenty-eight miles alone. Then Mark and Walter would alternate running with me the rest of the way, each doing three twelve-mile segments. The women would take turns in five-hour shifts, handing me food and drink and bringing me other aid as needed.

When the gun went off, the runners almost outnumbered the spectators. Eleven men and one woman started, ranging in age from sixteen to fifty-four. The temperature was 86°, dropping only to 70° during the night, and the relative humidity hovered near 100% for most of the run. There was no shade along the course and no breeze. The race director commented, "It's the worst day for running I've ever seen."

At the start my thoughts focused not on the weather or the distance, but on my right knee. Tendinitis of that knee had developed during the preceding month and had gotten much worse just before we were to leave Houston. I almost canceled the trip, but considering my year of intensive training, the plans all six of us had made, and opinions from two orthopaedic surgeons that the run would not permanently harm my knee, I decided to go ahead. As insurance, I began taking aspirin seven days before the race and took two tablets every four hours up to and throughout the run.

By the end of the first lap, I was drenched with sweat. This concerned and confused me because I had trained and raced for years in the brutal heat and humidity of Houston but had never sweated so profusely so early in a run. To complicate matters, a fine misty rain fell for the next four hours, making it impossible to judge the amount of my sweat loss. That, plus the heat, the humidity, and my painful knee, made the early part of the run unexpectedly hard for me. Nevertheless, I maintained a fairly steady pace of ten minutes a mile for the first forty miles. That pace included slowing down every four miles to drink, change glasses, towel off, and apply vaseline to chafe-prone areas. At twenty-eight miles Mark and Walter began taking turns running with me and did so unfalteringly for the remainder of the race. At about fifty miles, I noticed that my knee pain had disappeared and, from then on, I remained pain free.

From the very first I had to force myself to drink and, as the race progressed, the mere thought of drinking became more and more repulsive. This puzzled me because in all previous long runs on hot days I had craved and drunk a lot of fluid.

At sixty miles, about 3:30 in the morning, I became nauseated and sat down on the curb, unwilling and unable to drink my tea or ERG. Fortunately, Brenda located some bouillon. Two large cupfuls relieved my nausea considerably. Still, I had forty miles to go, and I was worried about the continuing effects of the heat and humidity.

When I had completed seventy miles, the 6,000 relay runners began stampeding by me. Each ran only four miles, but even some of them fell victim to the weather and were carted off in ambulances.

Between seventy and ninety miles, mental strain predominated. I hated everyone who had dreamed up four ultramarathon events and a massive relay race on the same course at the same time. I also resented the relay runners. Their task seemed miniscule compared with mine. They seemed to threaten bodily injury whenever they came whizzing by me, so I asked my partner to run directly behind me as a shield. Even my helpers irritated me whenever they tried to make me drink.

My sensory perception was distorted too. Every time my partner's foot struck a particular manhole cover, the clang startled and upset me. But the honking of cars, the noise of the crowd cheering the relay runners, the heat, the humidity, and my nagging nausea all seemed dulled by my obsessive concentration on finishing. At this point runners and spectators began to shout, "Hang in there, you're looking good." I thanked them for their encouragement, but I knew what I really looked like.

Around 8:30 in the morning, after eighty miles, I had a strong craving for the cookies I had brought, and I ate at least twenty. I washed them down with a cup of iced water, since I was afraid that any other liquid would make me vomit. My hunger abated, as did my lingering nausea, and I covered twelve more miles.

With only eight miles to go, heat illness struck me. The temperature had been climbing since dawn, and it was now noon. I suddenly became extremely nauseated and had to lie down because of dizziness. Noticing that I was pale and clammy, my helpers elevated my legs, covered me with cold, wet towels, and gave me ice to chew. They urged me to take fluids, but I couldn't drink anything. I didn't feel fatigued and had no muscle cramps or soreness, but for the first time during the run I questioned my ability to finish. (In retrospect, I believe that aspirin precipitated this heat illness.)

After fifteen minutes of being cooled down, I was able to continue with an ice-cold, wet towel draped over my head and shoulders, a cup of ice in hand, and both partners flanking me for moral support. Three times on this loop I doused myself with water from hoses supplied by people living along the route.

Still shaded by a cold, wet towel, I began the last four miles, Walter beside me. When the finish line came into view, he veered away, leaving me to run the last 300 yards alone. I had envisioned that moment many times during my training runs and throughout the race itself, fully expecting to swell with emotion. Instead, a constricting numbness engulfed me. With each succeeding step, I felt smaller and more insignificant.

At 2:20 in the afternoon, I crossed the finish line to the applause of my helpers and the race director. No one else was around. My time was 22:21:39. Of the 12 starters, 6 finished. Although I was the last to finish, it was the proudest moment of my life.

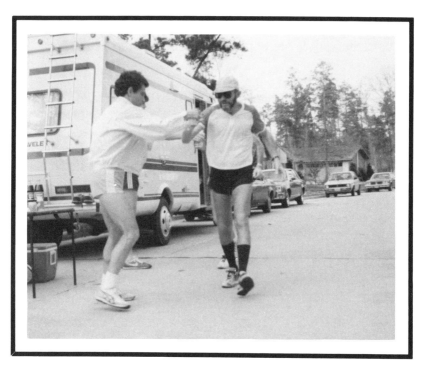

The author gets some aid on his way to setting national age (53) and age group (50–54) records for the 100-mile run (time: 17 hours, 2 minutes, 3 seconds), Houston, Texas, 19–20 February 1983. Note his two left arms and two right feet.

THE 100-MILE RUN: PREPARATION, PERFORMANCE, AND RECOVERY A CASE REPORT*

During 1978, some 1,060 runners entered ultramarathons in the United States.[1] That number is growing because more and more distance runners are seeking new challenges, and many are dissatisfied with the chaos typical of today's marathon.

The scientific literature is replete with data on the marathon but offers little information on ultramarathons and no specific study of the 100-mile run. This report summarizes my experiences with two 100-mile runs and correlates them with the experiences of eleven other runners who have raced that distance.

Case Report

In April 1966, I began a long-distance running program. By the end of 1969, I had logged almost 10,000 miles. During the next ten years, I ran an additional 58,118 miles, including thirty marathons, one 50-mile race, and two 100-km races.

*Reprinted by permission from the *American Journal of Sports Medicine* 1981; 9:258–61.

Preparation

I prepared for both of my 100-mile runs in much the same way. In the eleven months before the first race (May 1979) and the eight months before the second (February 1980), I averaged twenty miles per day at a pace of 8 to 10 minutes per mile. As the races neared, I did many 30-mile runs and one 40-mile run, tapering my mileage only in the final six days.

I craved and ate large amounts of meat, especially beef, with bran, fruit, and nuts for dessert. I also took one multivitamin tablet, 3 to 4 gm of vitamin C, and 4,000 IU of vitamin E daily, because that combination and dosage of vitamins seemed to keep me virtually free of muscle stiffness and soreness. Forty-eight hours before each race, I stopped eating all roughage. I also loaded up on animal protein and fat, because these foods seemed to boost my endurance.

Performance

The first run, the Primo 100-Mile Race, took place in Honolulu under miserably hot, humid conditions. Because I had tendinitis in my right knee, I took two aspirin tablets every four hours for a week before and *throughout* the run. That was a serious mistake, because the aspirin increased my sweating, urinary output, and body temperature while inhibiting my thirst. As a consequence, I felt sick all during the race and suffered severe heat exhaustion at ninety-two miles. After being covered with cold, wet towels for fifteen minutes, I was able to continue and finished the race in twenty-two hours, twenty-one minutes, thirty-nine seconds. My total fluid intake, despite prodigious fluid losses, was six quarts—only one-fourth of what I had planned to drink. My analysis of that race, with special reference to the adverse effects of aspirin, is the subject of another report.[2]

My second 100-mile run was in Houston. Freezing, windy conditions prevailed. Because I did not take any aspirin, and because of the weather, I lost much less fluid than in Honolulu. During the first forty miles, I drank two quarts of sugared tea. In the final sixty miles, I consumed one quart of water, two large packages of cookies, and 2.5 quarts of ice cream. In spite of the numbing cold, the run was surprisingly easy. I experienced none of the difficulties that I had in Honolulu, and I finished in nineteen hours, ten minutes, nineteen seconds.

Recovery

Recovery from the two runs differed. After the first one, I did not run for six days, and it took me a month to work up to my prerace mileage. After the second one, however, I resumed training the next day and, within a week, was running my usual twenty miles per day.

For one week after the first race, my lower legs and ankles were edematous. After the second race, similar swelling appeared, but it was milder and only lasted three days. Such swelling had not occurred previously. I had essentially no soreness after either run.

Methods

To put my experiences in perspective, I correlated them with information obtained by questionnaires from eleven other runners who have raced 100 miles. I also interviewed four of these runners. The questionnaires focused on the athletes' personal characteristics and running experiences, along with information related to their training technique, diet, vitamin intake, nourishment, and drug use during the 100-mile race, and their recovery thereafter.

Results

Table 1 lists the respondents according to age and presents relevant data from the questionnaires. Three women and nine men (including the author) made up the study group. They had been running from four to twenty-two years. Each had finished numerous marathons as well as one or more ultramarathons before attempting the 100-mile run.

Preparation

The training patterns varied considerably. Weekly mileage ranged from forty-two to 180, with five runners averaging ninety miles per week or less. Four (GD, DB, RA, and HF) trained only once per day; the remainder often trained twice per day. Three rested one or two days per week. Seven did speed work, usually once per week or less. Training pace, excluding speed work, ranged from seven to twelve minutes per mile, and most of the runners raced at approximately their training pace. The longest training run took place five days to eight weeks before the race and ranged from nineteen to sixty-two miles.

In preparing for the 100-mile run, four of the runners (LC, JB, DC, and GD) made no change in their training program. Two (MS and RA) made minimal changes in mileage and diet. The remainder, excluding the author, substantially increased their mileage (and in some cases their carbohydrate intake) six to twelve weeks before the race. I increased my mileage (and intake of animal protein) eleven months before the race.

The diets were all high in carbohydrates and most were low in fat. One respondent (MS) ate no animal protein; three (JB, PR, and DB) rarely ate animal protein; and at least one (HF) ate large amounts of animal protein.

Eight runners used vitamin C (0.5 to 6 gm), six used vitamin E (400 to 4,000 IU), and five used various combinations of the B vitamins daily. Some of them also used calcium, magnesium, zinc, iron, or desiccated liver.

In the final days before the race, all runners tapered their mileage. Most of them did not change their diet during this period, but two (MT and TK) loaded up on carbohydrates, and one (HF) loaded up on animal protein and fat. One (MS) fasted the day before the race.

Performance

All runners drank fluids at frequent intervals, typically every two to four miles, and in one case every half mile. The volume and type of fluid intake varied to some extent with the climatic conditions. Water, electrolyte replacement with glucose, fruit juice, sugared tea, and soup were the usual drinks. Six runners also consumed solid food, primarily in the latter stages of the run. They usually ate cookies, but some ate candy, fruit, ice cream, and even turkey sandwiches.

Use of aspirin during the run was detrimental. Two experienced hot-weather runners (PR and HF) took 10 grains of aspirin every four hours throughout the Honolulu race in May 1979, and both suffered heat exhaustion. In another race, one runner (DC) took two Tylenol tablets (McNeilab, Inc., Fort Washington, PA) every four hours without ill effects.

Difficulties during these races, apart from the two cases of heat exhaustion, were minimal. Some runners told of mental strain or fatigue; others mentioned minor muscle cramps early or late in the race; and one had gross hematuria.[3] None reported vomiting or diarrhea.

Recovery

Recovery was rapid. Some runners resumed training the next day, while others rested for up to eleven days. The majority reached prerace training levels within two weeks, and two began racing short distances by that time. Three runners (DC, GD, and HF) had edema in their lower legs or ankles, and one had a painful knee during the week after the race.

Discussion

This study demonstrates a wide variation in the ways athletes prepare for and run a 100-mile race. Moreover, the results suggest that an average marathoner can finish a 100-mile run without modifying his training program. Running shorter ultramarathons before attempting a 100-mile race is a logical step, but it probably does more to build confidence than to improve endurance.

Requisites for optimal performance in the 100-mile run remain ill defined. The data presented here show no consistent correlation between finishing times and a runner's age, sex, height, weight, running experience, weekly mileage, frequency and intensity of workouts, diet, use of vitamins and other supplements, or nourishment during the run.

Two variables that could influence the outcome of the race were not evaluated—the weather and the race course. Regarding the latter, RA volunteered the following: "My run was on a quarter-mile dirt track. That spared me the emotional stress of road hazards, traffic, dogs, confusing routes, etc. My aid and a restroom were only 440 yards away at any time and some other runner was always in view, if not running with me. The dirt surface cut down on body shock and was cooler than asphalt. Such factors will help in running 100 miles and in recovery." I would add that running at night along busy highways and dimly lit, winding streets—with no other runners in view and aid stations two miles apart—is indeed stressful.

One medically significant point in this investigation was that *aspirin is contraindicated if the run takes place in hot weather.* PR, a physician, confirmed my original findings about the detrimental effects of aspirin.[2] He took aspirin throughout the 1979 Primo Race to prevent or reduce anticipated musculotendinous discomfort. As the race progressed, his sweat losses increased and his thirst decreased. He finished with severe heat exhaustion. His performance in the 1978 Primo Race served as a control. That year he ran on the same course—for the same distance, and under the same climatic conditions—but did not take aspirin. He finished the race strongly. The amount of aspirin required to predispose the athlete to heat illness awaits clarification. Until such information becomes available, athletes would be wise not to combine aspirin with physical exertion in the heat.

Edema of the lower legs or ankles, as reported by three of the respondents, has been observed in other runners after ultramarathons.[4, 5] The cause of the edema is conjectural. I suspect that it is caused by a stress-induced rise in plasma levels of aldosterone and cortisol[6] with consequent sodium conservation and fluid retention.

Summary

This study analyzed the training methods and racing techniques of twelve athletes who have completed 100-mile runs. It showed that use of aspirin during the race can be dangerous if the run takes place in hot weather. No other consistent correlation was evident, however, between the variables examined and the finishing times. The findings suggest that an average marathoner can finish the 100-mile run without modifying his training program.

Addendum

From 21 to 22 February 1981 (in Houston, Texas), I ran 100 miles in eighteen hours, forty-five minutes, eleven seconds. This run differed from my previous 100-mile races in three respects. At the start, I had a head cold and generalized myalgia that disappeared during the run and did not recur. The weather was hot (71 to 78° F) and humid (58 to 76%) for the first fifty miles, then turned colder (55 to 61° F) with intermittent rain and winds up to 33 mph for the remainder of the race. Right-sided anterior tibial tendinitis, which developed at the seventy-mile mark and grew steadily more painful, slowed my pace accordingly. Because of the tendinitis, I could not resume running for eight days.

After submission of this paper, findings from a physiologic study of participants in a 100-mile track race have appeared in abstract form.[7, 8]

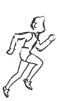

Acknowledgments

I am indebted to Ruth Anderson and to Jerome and Alice Tucker for their help in the early stages of this study.

TABLE 1
Data on 12 ultra-distance runners

Runner	Sex	Age (years)	Height (ft-in)	Weight (lb)	Occupation	Years of running	Weekly mileage	Speed work	Vitamins			Marathons		100-Mile runs[a]	
									B	C	E	Total	Best time (hr:min:sec)	Total	Best time (hr:min:sec)
MS	F	27	5-3	118	Saleswoman	13	100-140	−	+	+	+	30	3:14:52	2	19:03:00
CO	F	28	5-1	125	Secretary	6	125	+	+	+	−	10	3:39:04	1	19:27:46
LC	M	28	5-11½	133	Physician	16	55-60	+	−	−	−	33	2:33:45	1	13:33:46
JB	M	33	6-2	175	Law student	4	100	−	−	−	−	14	3:10:00	1	38:39:00
PR	M	34	6-0	175	Physician	16	120-180	+	−	+	+	10	2:52:00	2	14:42:59
MT	M	45	5-7	135	Airline representative	22	150	+	−	−	−	76	2:22:00	12	12:48:00
DC	M	46	5-11	180	Contractor	5	42	−	+	+	+	38	3:29:36	3	29:44:00
GD	M	46	5-9	145	Engineering professor	7	90	−	−	+	−	18	2:54:00	2	17:36:00
DB	M	46	6-1	142	Electrical assembler	5	80-85	+	−	+	+	10	3:07:00	2	20:23:00
TK	M	47	5-10	145	US Marine	7	105	+	−	−	−	23	3:12:00	5	17:56:26
RA	F	50	5-8	125	Nuclear chemist	7	55-60	+	+	+	+	40	3:04:19	1	16:50:47
HF	M	50	5-10½	150	Physician	14	130-160	−	+	+	+	30	3:08:23	2	19:10:19

[a]World road record = 11:51:11.

REFERENCES

[1]Hogan CL. Carousel of the mind. *Runner* 1980; 2:52–58.

[2]Fred HL. Reflections on a 100-mile run: Effects of aspirin therapy. *Med Sci Sports Exerc* 1980; 12:212–15.

[3]Fred HL. More on grossly bloody urine of runners. *Arch Intern Med* 1978; 138:1610–11.

[4]Gordon B, Baker JC. Observations on the apparent adaptability of the body to infections, unusual hardships, changing environment, and prolonged strenuous exertion. *Am J Med Sci* 1929; 178:1-8.

[5]Nakagome W, Hirayama T, Oka A, *et al.* Anthropometry of long distance race champions. *Jpn J Exp Med* 1932; 10:509–20.

[6]Newmark SR, Himathongkam T, Martin RP, *et al.* Adrenocortical response to marathon running. *J Clin Endocrinol Metab* 1976; 42:393–94.

[7]Phillips WH, Sucec AA, Selder DJ. Oxygen consumption and energy cost during ultramarathon running and walking performance. *Med Sci Sports Exerc* 1980; 12:87.

[8]Sucec AA, Phillips WH, Selder DJ. The effect of ultramarathon performance on maximal aerobic power and anaerobic threshold. *Med Sci Sports Exerc* 1980; 12:127.

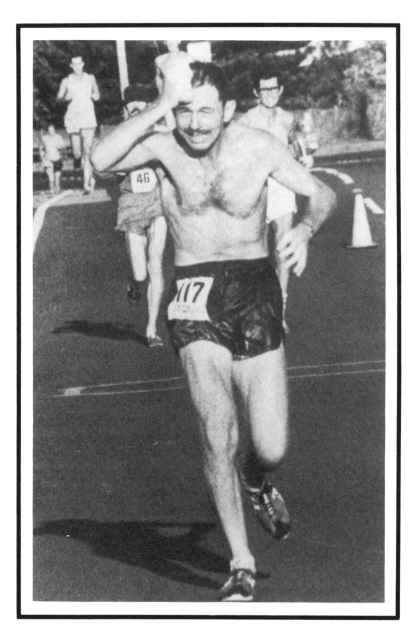

The author sponges off as he sweats out the Honolulu Marathon, Honolulu, Hawaii, 15 December 1974.

Aspirin for the Athlete— Friend or Foe?*

Warning: This drug can produce gastrointestinal ulceration and hemorrhage, delayed blood clotting, abdominal distress, nervous system disturbances, acid-base and electrolyte imbalances, hearing difficulty, liver damage, kidney malfunction, fever, asthma, and hives. Overdose may cause death from circulatory collapse and respiratory failure.

These precautions could be on the package insert required by the Food and Drug Administration if the product in question—aspirin—were new and being introduced for clinical use today.

Aspirin is a direct descendant of willow bark, which was known by the ancients to relieve pain and fever. The French chemist von Gerhardt first synthesized aspirin in 1853, but the compound remained on chemists' shelves for the next forty-five years.[6] It then became available for medicinal purposes as a powder and in 1915 entered the American market in tablet form.[16]

Aspirin is the world's most commonly used drug. In the United States alone, people ingest an estimated 50 million pounds of aspirin yearly,[1] an astonishing rate of about 100 million tablets daily. Moreover, aspirin is an ingredient in at

*Reprinted by permission from *Athletic Training* 1981; 202–203.

least 400 drug preparations[16] sold under various trade names. No wonder roughly 100,000 cases of serious and sometimes fatal aspirin poisoning occur each year.[1]

Certain symptoms should alert the user to the possibility of aspirin poisoning. Ringing in the ears is the most common first sign; others are dizziness, headache, confusion, weakness, nausea, and an increase in the depth and rate of respiration. These manifestations indicate that the dosage should be decreased or stopped completely.[1] Where is the dividing line between safe and unsafe usage of aspirin? A statistically safe dose is six tablets or less in 24 hours, with no more than two tablets in any four-hour period. This dosage should be taken for no more than three consecutive days. Even this "safe" amount, however, may cause gastrointestinal ulceration with consequent bleeding in at least half of those taking such quantity. Although the blood loss usually does not exceed a teaspoon a day, it could—if continued—result in iron-deficiency anemia and, in someone who already has a tendency to bleed easily, could be dangerous.

Aspirin can also affect bleeding in another way. As few as one to four tablets may delay the body's ability to clot blood.[16] Under normal conditions, this delay in blood clotting has little significance. But if the athlete then incurs an injury, the delayed clotting could lead to extensive hemorrhage into the damaged tissues.

When aspirin is taken on a continuing basis to relieve chronic discomfort, the chance of adverse reactions increases. So another warning deserves emphasis: *Therapeutic doses of aspirin (i.e., ten or more tablets daily for a week or more) should be taken only under the direction of a physician.*

Certain effects of aspirin—some good and some bad—have specific implications for the athlete. The good effects stem from the drug's well-known ability to reduce fever, relieve pain, and counteract inflammation. The bad effects relate to aspirin's poorly appreciated capacity to impair fluid balance by augmenting sweat losses, increasing urinary output, and inhibiting thirst.

Sweating is a characteristic response to aspirin intake when fever is present;[17] raised body temperature is a typicalconsequence of physical exertion;[10] and aspirin in large doses can even produce fever by increasing oxygen consumption and metabolism.[15] Thus, in hot weather, aspirin therapy may augment sweat losses, causing earlier and greater dehydration and higher body temperature than otherwise might be expected.

Increased urinary output is another potential outcome of aspirin therapy. Through its action on the kidneys, aspirin promotes excretion of sodium, potassium, glucose, and water.[11, 18]

How aspirin inhibits thirst awaits clarification. Current scientific knowledge suggests two mechanisms, one involving the brain[2, 8, 14] and the other, the kidneys.[3, 12, 13]

Considering these adverse effects, the author believes that aspirin can predispose athletes to heat illness. Two recently reported cases support this view.[4, 5] The amount of aspirin and the intensity and duration of exercise necessary for this reaction are not yet known. Until such information becomes available, athletes should use aspirin cautiously during competition in the heat.

One final precautionary note. Aspirin precipitates attacks of asthma, occasionally life-threatening, in a considerable proportion of known asthmatics and in a small percentage of the general population.[7, 16] Furthermore, athletes should be aware that the first symptoms of asthma may be wheezing and tightness in the chest that come on during or, more typically, shortly after physical exertion. Thus, athletes who have such symptoms (referred to as exercise-induced asthma) should scrupulously avoid aspirin and all proprietary mixtures containing it.[9]

If the athlete finds himself unable to tolerate aspirin, what are his alternatives? The choice depends upon the type of unfavorable reaction to aspirin and the ailment prompting use of the drug. When, for instance, the reaction is gastrointestinal bleeding, a buffered form of aspirin may eliminate it. For localized pain, applying heat, cold, or some other form of physical therapy may do the trick. But for generalized pain and for fever, acetaminophen (Tylenol, Datril, etc.) may be the answer. This nonprescription drug gives relief comparable to that of aspirin and is relatively safe in dosages of one or two tablets three or four times a day. Like aspirin, however, it should be taken for no more than several days at a time. Other medications such as Motrin and Indocin are effective as anti-inflammatory agents, but they require a prescription and have their own side effects.

Summary

Aspirin is a remarkably effective and inexpensive drug for reducing fever, relieving pain, and counteracting inflammation. Considering the frequency and amount of its use, aspirin is also remarkably safe. Nevertheless, its ability to produce serious adverse effects is substantial. If used sparingly and wisely, aspirin can be the athlete's friend. But if used without due respect for its harmful potential, aspirin can be the athlete's foe.

REFERENCES

[1]Cohen LS. Clinical pharmacology of acetylsalicylic acid. In Donoso E, Haft JI (Eds): *Thrombosis, Platelets, Anticoagulation, and Acetylsalicylic Acid.* New York, Stratton Intercontinental Medical Book Corporation, 1976.

[2]Epstein AM, Teitelbaum P. Severe and persistent deficits in thirst produced by lateral hypothalamic damage. In Wayner MJ (Ed): *Thirst,* pp. 395–410. New York, Macmillan Company, 1964.

[3]Flower RJ. Drugs which inhibit prostaglandin biosynthesis. *Pharmacol Rev* 1974; 26:33–67.

[4]Fred HL. Reflections on a 100-mile run: effects of aspirin therapy. *Med Sci Sports Exerc* 1980; 12:212–15.

[5]Fred HL. The 100-mile run: preparation, performance, and recovery. *Am J Sports Med* 1981; 9:258–61.

[6]Friend DG. Aspirin: the unique drug. *Arch Surg* 1974; 108:765–69.

[7]Gerhard H, Schachter EN. Exercise-induced asthma. *Postgrad Med* 1980; 67:91–102.

[8]Lascelles PT, Lewis PD. Hypodipsia and hypernatraemia associated with hypothalamic and suprasellar lesions. *Brain* 1972; 95:249–64.

[9]Leist ER, Banwell JG. Products containing aspirin. *N Engl J Med* 1974; 291:710–12.

[10]Maron MB, Horvath SM. The marathon: a history and review of the literature. *Med Sci Sports* 1978; 10:137–50.

[11]Rapoport S, Guest GM. The effect of salicylates on the electrolyte structure of the blood plasma. I. Respiratory alkalosis in monkeys and dogs after sodium and methyl salicylate; the influence of hypnotic drugs and of sodium bicarbonate on salicylate poisoning. *J Clin Invest* 1945; 24:759–69.

[12]Rogers PW, Kurtzman NA. Renal failure, uncontrollable thirst, and hyperreninemia; cessation of thirst with bilateral nephrectomy. *JAMA* 1973; 225:1236–38.

[13]Romero JC, Dunlap CL, Strong CG. The effect of indomethacin and other anti-inflammatory drugs on the reninangiotensin system. *J Clin Invest* 1976; 58:282–88.

[14]Smith MJH. Interactions with endocrine systems. In Smith MJH, Smith PK (Eds): *The Salicylates—A Critical Bibliographic Review,* pp. 116–25. New York, John Wiley and Sons, 1966.

[15]Smith PK. The pharmacology of salicylates and related compounds. *Ann N Y Acad Sci* 1960; 86:38–63.

[16]Weiss HJ. Aspirin—a dangerous drug? *JAMA* 1974; 229:1221–22.

[17]Woodbury DM. Analgesics and antipyretics: salicylates and congeners; phenacetin and congeners; antipyrine and congeners; colchicine. In Goodman LS, Gilman A (Eds): *The Pharmacological Basis of Therapeutics, 3rd Edition,* p. 314. New York, Macmillan Company, 1965.

[18]Woodbury DM. Analgesics and antipyretics: salicylates and congeners; phenacetin and congeners; antipyrine and congeners; colchicine. In Goodman LS, Gilman A (Eds): *The Pharmacological Basis of Therapeutics, 3rd Edition,* p. 319. New York, Macmillan Company, 1965.

OBSERVATIONS
(MEDICAL AND OTHERWISE)
FROM THE TRANS-TEXAS RACE*

After five stages and 258 miles, I can't move my left foot up or down. Tendinitis has brought me to a standstill. I wait three days, and still I can barely walk, much less run. Greatly disappointed, I withdraw from the Sesquicentennial Trans-Texas Race.

Back home, I tell myself repeatedly that it was the best thing for me to do, my only sensible option. But my heart remains with the runners, and I keep thinking about the week I spent with them. So, as I await news of their progress, I relive that week from two perspectives: physician and runner.

Medical Observations

Though I enter this race solely as a participant, I'm also the only M.D. on the scene. Consequently, most of the medical problems come to my attention.

(1) Swelling of the feet and ankles appears by the second day in about half of the competitors, including me. In some, the swelling progresses and becomes painful, prompting its victims to loosen laces and cut out the toes of their shoes.

*Reprinted by permission from *Ultrarunning* 1987; January-February:12–14.

Unfortunately, that approach can't solve my problem. I'm wearing Sock Trainers, a shoe I had logged thousands of miles in without the predicament I now face—extreme pressure and growing pain over the midfoot, near the ankle. Unbuckling the midfoot support strap doesn't help. The culprit is the constricting fit of the nylon stretch material. Slitting the material at the ankle or over the midfoot simply shifts the pressure point toward the toes. By the time I try another shoe, it's too late.

Tendinitis has developed, and my feet and ankles are so swollen that I have to remove my full-length orthotics to get my shoes on. But I can't run very far without orthotics— the chance of a lifetime is slipping away. In fairness to the Sock Trainers, the lead runner is wearing them (but without orthotics). He also tells me that in a previous 1,000-mile race, he started in a size ten shoe of another make but needed a size thirteen to finish.

What accounts for the swelling of our feet and ankles? Several possibilities come to mind. First, and most likely, is a decrease in urinary excretion of sodium with resultant sodium retention and subsequent fluid accumulation. This conservation of sodium, mediated by the hormone aldosterone, represents the body's attempt to counterbalance the fluid losses, electrolyte changes, and reduced kidney blood flow associated with strenuous, protracted exercise. Other factors that may contribute to the swelling are tissue damage from the cumulative effect of pounding the concrete and asphalt, and pooling of fluid from long hours in the upright position. I wonder, too, whether the swelling itself causes further swelling by impairing venous and lymphatic drainage from the foot.

(2) Tendinitis affects five of us. In my case, intense inflammation of the big tendon on top of the left foot (extensor hallucis longus), the tendon at the ankle (extensor digitorum longus), and the major tendon in front of the shin (anterior tibial) sidelines me. The pain, swelling, and crepitation take ten days to subside.

The other four runners have Achilles tendinitis, bilateral in three and unilateral in one. Three of them split the heels of their shoes; this reduces pressure around the Achilles and gives relief. The other just loosens his shoe laces. All four continue.

Tendons of the foot and ankle presumably get squeezed as our feet get bigger and our shoes get tighter. In turn, the squeezing impedes free movement of the tendons within their sheaths, leading to further irritation and swelling. Continued running for unusually long distances—especially over hard surfaces whose slant and grade are frequently changing—definitely aggravates and may be the prime cause of the condition.

(3) Swelling of the knees crops up in two runners within seventy-two hours. In one, the swelling is bilateral, minimal, slightly tender, and fleeting. In the other, however, it is unilateral, massive, painless, and persistent. Both runners are still going when I quit.

The genesis of this swelling is speculative. Both runners have concomitant bilateral Achilles tendinitis, which may alter their normal running style, thereby increasing the strain on their involved knees.

(4) Eyelid swelling is striking; we all look like bees have stung us. At first I think that running directly into freezing rain and strong wind is the explanation. Our hands and forearms are swollen, too, and initially I assume that it's because our arms are hanging down most of the time. But then I notice that the swelling persists after the weather improves and that lying down doesn't reduce it. I suspect, therefore, that the swelling is primarily a consequence of the sodium retention mentioned previously. My own eyes, hands, and forearms do not return to normal until three days after I stop running. This lag may represent the time it takes for kidney function and hormonal activity to return to normal once the exertion ends.

(5) Muscle ailments are generally mild and inconsequential. Although we all have fatigue and stiffness at the end of each run, our zip and flexibility surprisingly return every morning. One runner, however, suffers stiffness, pain, and swelling of the muscles and connective tissues (myofasciitis) on one side of his back. I ascribe this to the way he positions his shoulders and swings his arms.

(6) Miscellaneous afflictions include hypothermia in three runners, blistered feet in two, food poisoning in two, infected toes in one, and a possible stress fracture of the foot in one.

Some of these observations intrigue me, and I hope to follow up on them when the race is over.

The Race

Inept planning, pitiful organization, woefully deficient support services, unfulfilled promises, and miscommunication mar this race, creating inexcusable hardships for the runners and volunteers. If this sounds like sour grapes, read on.

(1) From day one, the most support we ever have consists of three commercial vans, one motor home, and two to four volunteers—in shocking contrast to what we expect. "You don't have to bring a handler," the prerace information sheet says. "Few handlers can take care of you as well as the Texas National Guard. Due to their involvement, this is likely to be the best organized and supported race of its size in history." The fact is, only two guardsmen ever show up, and they disappear after one and two days, respectively.

(2) Each stage is too far to cover in daylight, so we run at night—some literally all night long. And worse—much worse—we have absolutely no protection against the traffic. We discover that running or walking along the narrow shoulders of major highways, with or against traffic and particularly without any protection, is harder and more dangerous than we had thought. You can't afford to stumble, weave, or lose your concentration because one misstep can

be your last. Wind gusts from passing eighteen-wheelers blow you off your feet and deposit you five yards down the way. Your eyes play tricks on you. You think you see a support van, but it turns out to be a bush. You think you see a sign, but it turns out to be an oncoming truck. Getting lost is a continuous possibility, and two runners do so. These difficulties and the threat of being injured or killed multiply exponentially at night. I plead for a cut-off time at dark. The plea fails.

(3) The dismal support system forces some runners to go hours without nourishment or a much-needed change of clothes. Four runners pick up the slack by spending much of the day (or night) driving the vans. I am fortunate. My wife Judy and my son, Mike, use my car and serve as my aides. They also offer help to the other runners when they can.

(4) Mile markers are absent, and the support vehicles are either too spread out on the course or too often deployed elsewhere to assist us in this regard. This keeps us guessing as to how far we've gone and how far we still have to go. Especially disturbing is finding out late in a run that the scheduled distance for that day has been increased, sometimes up to eight miles.

(5) Transferring from the finish line each night to where we're supposed to sleep is an ordeal. There aren't enough vans to transport each runner to the motel room soon after he finishes. Consequently, runners must wait, sometimes for three hours, until the van is full. The subsequent travel to the motel may take an additional hour. Getting from the motel back to the previous finish line to start the next day's run may take an hour, too. This wasted motion exhausts us and frustrates us. And on top of our attempts to run fifty-plus miles a day, it leaves little time to bathe, eat, or sleep. We also have no time to wash or dry our gear, and everybody around us "nose" it.

(6) "We've . . . arranged for free sleeping facilities every night" the prerace information sheet says. Not true. No one seems to know until the last minute whether we have any place to sleep, and if we do, where and what kind it is. And one night we have to locate and pay for our own lodging.

(7) Getting enough food is another concern. Breakfast is not always obtainable, and finding a place for dinner is a hassle at best. There is no time to buy groceries, and the supplements furnished during the runs are meager by anyone's standards.

(8) There is no official medical supervision. And, so far as we know, medical supplies are not available. One runner uses a toothpick from a hamburger to puncture a blister.

On day eight, the thirteen runners and that day's volunteers hold a meeting to discuss the mess we're in. No one in the room and no one since the race began admits to being the race director. We contact the moguls in Houston who have been calling the shots, but they know nothing about the support a run of this type requires. They obviously don't understand our plight and don't seem to care. Furthermore, we get no assurance that our lot will improve. "We're just pawns in a public relations chess game," one runner says. Another replies, "It won't be who wins, but who survives. And whoever does survive will do so despite, not because of, the (non)help he gets." We all feel betrayed and resentful.

The continued disregard for our safety and welfare persuades four runners to withdraw. It also erases my lingering desire to re-enter the run, so I leave too.

The runners should be nearing Houston now, and my excitement and concern for them are building. How many are left? What condition are they in? Did their support get better? I'll know soon.

Epilogue

About the time the race ended, I examined Emile, Scott, Jack, and Doyle; interviewed Clarence; and obtained reliable information on Bob:

(1) Emile had nagging Achilles tendinitis and inflamed back muscles throughout the run. During the final three stages, he also had flagrant right-sided anterior tibial and extensor digitorum longus tendinitis. But nothing slowed him down. Il est magnifique!

(2) Bob's only problems were blistered feet and lack of sleep. Six days after the race, he covered 114 miles in a forty-eight-hour run. A "Wise" man once said, "Walk, don't run."

(3) Clarence shrugged off hypothermia and blisters and was otherwise unscathed. "Would I were steadfast as thou art—" (Keats).

(4) Scott overcame early ankle pains and several bouts of hypothermia, gathered steam as the race progressed, and finished strong. Six days later, he completed 164 miles during a forty-eight-hour run. Great Scott!

(5) Jack triumphed over infected toes and was in second place, performing brilliantly, when right-sided anterior tibial tendinitis halted him just five stages short of smelling the roses. Damn.

(6) Doyle, close behind Jack, succumbed in the same stage to left-sided anterior tibial and extensor digitorum longus tendinitis. The massive swelling of his left knee had resolved during the second week, some 400 miles after it developed. Incredible!

All but one of these competitors were puffy-eyed and thick fingered when they finished, but their eyes and hands returned to normal three to four days thereafter.

Carlos's lamentable accident, a hit-and-run at night, crushed his left upper arm, splintering the bone and disrupting the nerves and blood vessels. To date, he has undergone three operations, including bone, nerve, and vein grafts to the affected site. He remains hospitalized.

Finally, the runners and a volunteer told me that the support services did not improve substantially during the second and third weeks of the run.

Conclusions

(1) Participants in multiday races would do well to bring along extra shoes larger than those they ordinarily wear.

(2) Tendinitis may be the injury most likely to stop a runner in such races.

(3) In the planning and development of any staged, multiweek race, experienced ultradistance runners should have the controlling say-so. Equally important is having an

experienced ultradistance runner as the clearly designated, full-time, on-the-spot race director with the authority to modify the run as common sense dictates.

(4) Footraces on U.S. thoroughfares, no matter how well organized or supported, carry an inordinate amount of risk to life and limb. Therefore, if such races must take place, they should be conducted in daylight only.

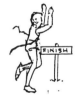

Freezing rain, gale-force winds, and speeding eighteen-wheelers harass the author as he plods endlessly down U.S. Highway 87—as seen through the wet windshield of his handler's car.